Practice
Management
Module

Ambulatory
Care

**CLINICAL
SKILLS
PROGRAM**

American Society of Health-System Pharmacists

Any correspondence regarding this publication should be sent to the publisher, American Society of Health-System Pharmacists®, 7272 Wisconsin Avenue, Bethesda, MD 20814, attn: Jane S. Ricciuti, Pharmacist Editor/ Project Manager, Special Publishing. Produced in conjunction with the ASHP Publications Production Center (Bill Fogle, Technical Editor).

The information presented herein reflects the opinions of the contributors and reviewers. It should not be interpreted as an official policy of ASHP or as an endorsement of any product.

Drug information and its applications are constantly evolving because of ongoing research and clinical experience and are often subject to professional judgment and interpretation by the practitioner and to the uniqueness of a clinical situation. The author and ASHP have made every effort to ensure the accuracy and completeness of the information presented in this book. However, the reader is advised that the publisher, author, contributors, editors, and reviewers cannot be responsible for the continued currency of the information, for any errors or omissions, and/ or for any consequences arising from the use of the information in the clinical setting.

The reader is cautioned that ASHP makes no representation, guarantee, or warranty, express or implied, that the use of the information contained in this book will prevent problems with insurers and will bear no responsibility or liability for the results or consequences of its use.

ISBN: 1-879907-92-5

Contents

Preface

Pharmacists practicing in ambulatory care settings are increasingly responsible for designing, recommending, and managing patient-specific pharmacotherapy regimens. Patients in an ambulatory care setting usually present with chronic conditions; thus, pharmacists in this setting develop long-term relationships with patients. An important element of this care is creating a pharmacy practice setting that fosters this pharmacist-patient relationship. Another key element is establishing an environment that reinforces the collaborative relationship between pharmacists and other health care professionals.

The *Ambulatory Care Clinical Skills Program: Practice Management Module* covers content areas needed to launch an ambulatory care pharmacy practice: creating a business plan, designing the care facility, complying with laboratory regulations, marketing, documenting, and seeking reimbursement for patient care services.

Writers

MedOutcomes, Inc.

Wendy Munroe Rosenthal, Pharm.D.
Geneva Clark Briggs, Pharm.D., BCPS
Thomas Rosenthal

Contributors

ASHP wishes to acknowledge the following people who contributed their time and expertise to the development of this text:

Angela Aldrich
Sandra Oh Clarke
Michelle A. Fritsch
Peter Gal
Leslie Dotson Jaggers
Viktoria Kharlamb
Peter Koval
Con Ann Ling
Jennifer Lofland
Jennifer Wilson Norton
Lisa Oliver
Cynthia Reilly
Jane S. Ricciuti
Mary Anne Roark
Terry Rubin
Marie A. Smith
Kathleen A. Snella

Introduction

Who Can Benefit From Using the *Practice Management Module?*

ASHP created the *Ambulatory Care Clinical Skills Program: Practice Management Module* as part of a profession-wide effort to increase pharmacy's involvement in clinical practice and pharmaceutical care in the ambulatory care setting. Both pharmacists and pharmacy students can enhance their business and management skills by engaging in these self-study activities. Staff pharmacists, pharmacy managers and directors, recent graduates, and pharmacy students can benefit from this program, working either alone or as part of a curricular or staff development plan.

The Best Way to Use the Clinical Skills Program

When using the *Ambulatory Care Clinical Skills Program: Practice Management Module*, you can either work alone or as part of a group. If you are working alone, you may want to ask your practice site supervisor to help you practice the skills you learn.

The units of the *Ambulatory Care Clinical Skills Program: Practice Management Module* should be studied in sequential order. The *Ambulatory Care Clinical Skills Program: Practice Management Module* is a carefully structured, systematic approach to establishing a pharmacy practice setting.

How to Study

Successful completion of this self-study module may require that you adopt some different approaches than those you customarily use for classroom learning. If you have never used a self-study text before, you will quickly discover that learning can be difficult when you do not have a teacher answering your questions, demonstrating the relationships between ideas, setting deadlines, or evaluating your work. A good self-instruction program guides you through the text as if a teacher were presenting the material and supplies you with study aids. Make this module an effective self-study tool by following these suggestions:

1. Set a goal for completing the module and establish a schedule for studying without interruption or distraction. A library may be an ideal place for this project.

2. Read the introduction and learning objectives of each unit. These sections will tell you why the unit is important, what specific information you will be expected to learn for answering the self-study questions, and how the unit is organized.

3. Scan the unit, noting the subject headings.

4. Read the unit, keeping the learning objectives in mind. Underline or highlight important passages and make notes in the margins.

5. Read the summary to review the main points of the unit. Review anything that still seems unclear.

6. Answer the self-study questions to evaluate your understanding of the information.

7. Review information pertaining to the questions that you answered incorrectly.

Module Organization

The *Ambulatory Care Clinical Skills Program: Practice Management Module* is divided into 12 units. You should study these units in the order presented because each unit builds on understanding gained from the prior unit. Each unit begins with an introduction explaining the relevance of what you will learn, the objectives you will attain, and the organizational structure of the material. At the end of each unit summary are self-study questions you can use to check your mastery of the objectives.

Getting Started

UNIT 1

To be successful in the ambulatory patient care environment, you need not only clinical skills but also a practice environment that supports the provision of service. The combination of clinical expertise and a supportive environment is established through practice management. There are many elements of practice management that must be considered when establishing or expanding ambulatory patient care services. For the purposes of this book, *ambulatory patient care services* is defined as direct pharmaceutical care services provided to patients in an outpatient environment, exclusive of dispensing services.

Unit 1 will review issues that require initial decisions. These issues include potential roles for the pharmacist in an ambulatory care setting, assessment of your setting, and implementation and management planning. The elements that will be discussed in subsequent units include facility design; establishing a laboratory; setting up systems for making appointments, for ordering and tracking patient education materials, and for tracking patients; documentation; screening services; marketing; legal issues; quality care provision; and reimbursement for services.

Unit Objectives

After you successfully complete this unit, you will be able to:
- describe the potential roles of pharmacists in ambulatory patient care services,
- describe how the assessment of services affects the establishment of an ambulatory patient care practice, and
- describe the role of business and operational plans in establishing ambulatory patient care services.

Unit Organization

This unit describes initial decisions in establishing or expanding ambulatory patient care services. It begins with a discussion of possible roles of pharmacists in the ambulatory patient care setting. Next, you will learn factors that are used to determine the scope of practice, including an assessment of services. Finally, you will learn how business and operational plans are used to increase the likelihood of success.

The Role of Pharmacists in Various Ambulatory Care Settings

There is tremendous potential for pharmacists in the ambulatory care setting as more and more medical care moves from an acute care to an outpatient setting. Currently, the role of pharmacists in the ambulatory care setting is varied and continues to expand. A major role for ambulatory care pharmacists is to assume responsibility for patients' pharmacotherapeutic and related health care problems and complementing the patient goals of other health care professionals (e.g., physicians and dietitians). Some of the functions performed by pharmacists in ambulatory care settings are listed in **Table 1**.

The functions an individual pharmacist performs will vary with the setting. In some cases, pharmacists may be generalists who work with patients with many different conditions and perform both direct patient care activities, such as individualizing therapeutic regimens, and administrative functions, such as designing prescription drug benefits for insured patients. Other ambulatory care pharmacists specialize in particular disease states or drug therapy. Some of the more common specialty areas include anticoagulation, diabetes, asthma, hypertension, and hyperlipidemia. Some of the less common specialty areas are weight control, smoking cessation, infertility, and congestive heart failure. Specialized pharmacists tend to perform more patient care activities and fewer administrative activities.

Assessment of Services

In defining your scope of practice it is important to detail the nature and extent of patient care services you will offer and to anticipate potential problems and address them proactively. For example, imagine you are operating a weight loss clinic and during the routine initial screening of a patient you recognize that he is experiencing signs and symptoms suggestive of diabetes. In this case, you must have a clear understanding of the scope of your practice and how to refer this patient for care. Another example would be establishing the service levels for an anticoagulation clinic. Will the clinic offer on-call, 24-hour service and, if not, how will emergency

Table 1. Pharmacist Functions in Ambulatory Care Settings

Patient Care Activities

Identify pharmacotherapeutic and related health care problems.

Establish desired pharmacotherapeutic goals for each pharmacotherapeutic and related health care problem.

Design monitoring plans to determine whether the desired therapeutic goal has been achieved.

Individualize therapeutic regimens.

Determine the most cost-effective therapeutic plan.

Participate in multidisciplinary teams to provide care.

Coordinate health services and promote continuity of care through collaboration with other health care providers, the patient, and the family.

Support the patient and the family.

Make appropriate recommendations for therapy or referrals to other health care providers.

Have authority to modify medication dosages or order laboratory tests.

Provide oral counseling about medications.

Provide written information about medications.

Provide oral and written information about patient's disease states.

Monitor patient outcomes.

Conduct wellness and prevention programs.

Monitor medication regimen adherence.

Administrative Activities

Develop clinical practice or disease management guidelines.

Conduct medication management programs (drug use review [DUR] or medication use evaluation [MUE]).

Seek reimbursement for services.

Conduct academic detailing.

Provide physician profiles or report cards.

Negotiate pharmaceutical contracts.

Make decisions for large populations on the basis of pharmacoepidemiology.

Design pharmaceutical benefits.

Collect HEDIS (Health Plan Employer Data and Information Set) data.

Use pharmacoeconomic data for formulary decision-making.

Create economic and clinical outcomes reports.

Combination Activities

Track adverse drug reactions.

Identify patients/providers who use medications inappropriately.

Work to change behavior of individual patients and providers.

Source: references 1–3.

service be provided and the necessary access procedure be communicated to patients? These scope-of-practice issues dictate the resources and staff competence necessary to serve patients effectively.

No matter what the setting, the pharmacist's focus is patient care activities. The extent of individual involvement varies from site to site. In general, involvement in administrative activities varies much more among settings than patient care activities do. In the community/retail setting, pharmacists are less likely to be involved in policy and formulary enforcement activities and some of the other administrative activities listed in **Table 1**. They may be more involved in seeking reimbursement for services and dealing with day-to-day business decisions. In the HMO setting, pharmacists may be more involved in administrative activities but, depending on the financial arrangements for the setting, are less likely to deal with reimbursement issues. In the clinic setting, depending on the funding structure, pharmacists may be involved in seeking reimbursement for their services. Whether the clinic is part of a health system or is an independent site usually determines whether the pharmacist is involved in policy and formulary enforcement and development.

Examine the roles you can have in your setting. Once you have done this, you can then visualize what services you could offer that incorporate these roles. For example, suppose that you are a dispensing pharmacist in the community-based pharmacy of a hospital/health system in a large metropolitan area. Recently, your health system has been increasing the percentage of patients for whom reimbursement is capitated. Many of your diabetic patients are followed at a diabetes clinic at the hospital. You recognize that a large percentage are not adhering to their prescribed medication therapy and are not keeping their scheduled appointments at the clinic. Your vision is to offer outpatient services at your location, which is more convenient to your patient population. You are confident you can increase adherence to self-monitoring and medication therapy, thereby reducing patient readmittance to the hospital and emergency room visits.

Building a Business Plan

You should think of patient care service in the ambulatory care setting as a business. Before establishing a patient care service you must create a business plan, knowing that garnering all of the

resources to make your vision a reality will require convincing other people to support your ideas. A business plan will help you organize your thoughts, avoid overlooking issues, and provide a clear set of long-term objectives. It will help you focus on the activities involved in establishing and sustaining the program. Business plans may be simple or complex, but they require that you do a global assessment to identify:

- potential clients for your services and their unmet needs,
- the purpose of the business (goals),
- skills and interests of staff,
- competition,
- the services offered by the business,
- the customers of the business (in addition to payers), and
- the realistic financial goals and market potential of the business.

Potential clients for your services may include patients, health insurers (i.e., managed care organizations, traditional insurers, and government programs such as Medicare and Medicaid), and employers who bear the cost of their employees' health care coverage. Successful partnering with a payer for the provision of pharmaceutical care requires you to identify an unmet need on their part that is resolved by your services. For example, you could provide a program to improve medication regimen adherence in a target population of patients who incur high costs or are high utilizers of health services. This approach will appeal to many health care insurers, who tend to focus on what can be done to reduce the health care costs of outlying patient populations.

Any patient care service offered must be a high-quality, consistent service and must achieve measurable outcomes that are favorable. The health care marketplace requires performance. As is true with all businesses, no one is paying for hard work; they are paying for positive outcomes. This foundational concept must be considered when designing and developing your service.

Program evaluation will be measured by the outcomes achieved with the patients. If program services are not matched with staff competences, the opportunity for failure is very high. You should assess your and your staff's personal skills and interests. This will determine what services you are currently able to provide and which would require additional training or staff to provide.

You may need to adapt the services you plan to offer to avoid competing with other professionals within your setting. This will help you avoid internal conflicts. For example, if your setting has a dietitian, nurse practitioner, and exercise physiologist, your services should complement rather than compete with the services those professionals provide. This is not to say that you may not want to compete with professionals providing similar services outside your setting. If you feel you cannot offer a service unique enough to overcome the competition outside your setting, you may wish to look for another area to pursue.

To determine what services to offer, identify the goals of your program and then determine what services you must provide to achieve those goals. Identify what services would most interest the decision-makers in your setting. To sell your services to management and/or payers, your initial role may be narrowly focused to get that first approval. The ultimate goal of your services may be totally different from your initial goal. Your goals may have several different levels. For example, in an integrated health care setting, you may initially be able to persuade management to allow you to set up patient care clinics based on cost containment (i.e., medication cost reductions through changing and improving physician prescribing behavior). The next goal may be to decrease hospitalizations and the length of stay when patients are hospitalized. Finally, your goal may be to improve clinical outcomes, such as having 90% of diabetic patients within an accepted range for a physiological measure, such as hemoglobin A_{1c}.

You need to identify the primary customers of your services for marketing efforts. This will be discussed further in unit 8. Some of the customers of your services may include patients, physicians, payers, and the managers of your setting.

Because patient care services are a business, you need to identify the financial goals and market potential for your services. You need to forecast revenues, including the source of the funds, even if they are an expansion of a current budget line or reductions in costs from other areas. For example, the establishment of an anticoagulation clinic is expected to result in decreased hospitalizations. The decreased number of days of expected hospitalizations multiplied by the variable cost of a hospital day will produce an expected savings that can be shown as revenue for your service. For example, in a population of 100 patients on anticoagulation therapy, you reduced patient hospitalizations by 4.

At your institution, the average hospital stay is 5 days, so you have avoided 20 days. If the average variable cost for the hospital is $750 per day, then the overall savings you achieved is $15,000.

All of the costs of the program must be projected, which allows you to determine a bottom line. A financial analysis of relevant financial indicators (e.g., return on investment) can then be calculated.

For example, imagine that you are in a community pharmacy setting and wish to begin a patient care service. You have a strong interest in diabetes and have completed a certificate training program in diabetes care. You have noticed that many of your patients with diabetes appear to have problems with medication regimen adherence, and frequent hospitalizations result. Because there is not a structured program for patients with diabetes offered in your community, you decide to implement a diabetes management service. The potential payers for your service include the patients and their insurers and employers. The purposes of the program may include helping patients take their medications appropriately to decrease adverse events, attracting new patients (customers) to your pharmacy, and providing new revenue for the pharmacy. The services you plan to offer may include medication monitoring and management, patient education, laboratory monitoring, and feedback to patients' other health care providers. The customers for your new service are persons with diabetes who currently use your pharmacy and those who do not, as well as physicians who may refer patients to you. Your financial goal for the program may be to break even the first year and show a modest profit the second year. The market potential of the business depends on the number of persons with diabetes in your service area and on your competition.

Here is another example of an analysis of relevant financial indicators. Imagine that you work for an HMO and have been asked to develop some strategies to reduce medication costs and hospitalizations among certain populations. Based on analyses done by the finance department, a large number of the HMO's high-cost patients have asthma. You have staff with training in asthma, so you decide to open an asthma management clinic. The HMO is the payer in this case because it is absorbing the cost of running the clinic, based on the assumption it will save money for the HMO. The clinic's purpose will be to contain medication costs, hospitalizations, and emergency room visits among a select group of patients. The clinic will provide medication monitoring and management, medication initiation and dosage adjustments, and patient education. Although management will identify a list of problematic patients for the clinic to target, the clinic's primary customers will be the physicians who must approve their patients' enrollment. Based on a financial analysis of potential cost savings, one financial goal will be to decrease resource utilization by 25% the first year. The market potential may be limited initially because the service will be provided to a select group of patients. If successful, this clinic has the potential for expansion, and its success would justify the development of clinics to target other patient populations and conditions.

Operational Plan

Your business plan should include a section that addresses how you will operate the services to increase the likelihood that your efforts will produce the desired outcomes. Pharmaceutical care requires capable pharmacists, sufficient resources, and support from all personnel of the organization in which it is practiced. Its delivery is impossible without the cooperation of pharmacy managers who understand it, are committed to it, and will create a system that facilitates it.

Pharmacy managers must not only ensure that pharmacists are well educated about the practice of pharmaceutical care; they must also develop an environment wherein pharmaceutical care can be effectively, efficiently, and economically practiced. They have to put the structure together to let people work. The successful delivery of pharmaceutical care requires an organization to have an operational plan that:

- has a mission statement to reflect the commitment to pharmaceutical care;
- has a set of specific goals for all participants in the program, including, but not limited to, patients, pharmacists, physicians, and clients;
- clearly defines the work to be completed by the pharmacist and support personnel;
- clearly defines the standard of practice and includes evaluation criteria for job performance;
- has an organizational structure that supports the work defined (including job descriptions that accurately state the responsibilities to be accomplished and the experience, skills, and knowledge needed to accomplish them);

- creates a quality assurance monitoring program that will provide feedback on competence;
- provides opportunity for continuing education for staff;
- defines the proper financial systems with adequate internal controls;
- clearly defines an outcomes monitoring program, including patient clinical outcomes and the program's financial status;
- assigns responsibilities for all tasks to specific individuals; and
- has timelines for the completion of all tasks.

Summary

Before implementing patient care services, you need to assess the roles you have in your setting and then create a business plan that establishes the need for your program and identifies how you can solve the problems through your services, which are likely to be accepted by the setting and reimbursed. There are many books and software products available that will assist in the development of an effective business plan that will make a strong and compelling case for the implementation of patient care services. Communicating and selling your business plan can require perseverance and flexibility. Use your business plan to secure supporters of the program who will aid you in your quest for acceptance.

Once you determine what services you plan to offer, establish an operational plan to ensure smooth start-up and operation of your services. With well-designed business and operational plans, you increase your chance of success in this endeavor.

References

1. Plein, JB. Pharmacy's paradigm: welcoming the challenges and realizing the opportunities. *Am J Pharm Ed* 1992;56:283–7.

2. [Anonymous]. Paper from the Commission to Implement Change in Pharmaceutical Education: Maintaining our commitment to change. *Am J Pharm Ed* 1996;60:378–84.

3. American Society of Health-System Pharmacists (ASHP), Center on Managed Care Pharmacy. *Survey of Managed Care and Ambulatory Care Pharmacy Practice in Integrated Health Systems.* Bethesda, MD: ASHP; 1997.

Self-Study Questions

Objective

Describe the potential roles of pharmacists in ambulatory patient care services.

1. State the functions that pharmacists can perform in ambulatory care settings.

2. Describe how specialization might affect the functions that a pharmacist performs.

Objective

Describe how the assessment of services affects the establishment of an ambulatory patient care practice.

3. Which of the following best describes how the scope of practice is determined?

    A. You should focus on patients who will reimburse your practice for services because this is the primary determinant of success.

    B. It is not important to determine the needs of patients in your area because patients will be referred to your practice.

    C. You should determine the roles and skills of existing staff, as well as the needs and wants of potential clients and patients.

    D. You should offer services similar to those offered by other health care professionals in your setting to stimulate competition.

4. Determining the scope of services helps you to do all of the following *except*:

    A. identify potential problems before they occur.

    B. determine the need for emergency services.

    C. determine staff education and training needs.

    D. determine fees to charge for services.

Objective

Describe the role of business and operational plans in establishing ambulatory patient care services.

5. Potential clients for ambulatory patient care services include:

    A. patients.

    B. managed care organizations.

    C. Medicare.

    D. All of the above are potential clients.

6. Explain how service and financial goals of a business plan may change over time.

7. Describe the purpose of an operational plan.

Self-Study Answers

1. Pharmacists may perform patient care, administration, or a combination of these activities.

2. Pharmacists in specialty areas of practice (e.g., diabetes and asthma management) may perform more direct patient care than administrative functions.

3. C

4. D

5. D

6. Initial service goals may focus on cost containment in order to convince management to provide services. Later goals may focus more on patient outcomes. Financial goals for the first year may be to break even, whereas goals for successive years may be to increase profit.

7. An operational plan creates an environment that increases a facility's likelihood of success by fostering pharmaceutical care.

Facility Design

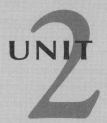

Providing pharmaceutical care in the ambulatory care setting requires an environment that is conducive to private pharmacist-patient interaction. A private setting fosters a relaxed and confidential atmosphere that facilitates communication. Putting patients in the proper frame of mind to discuss their health concerns promotes development of a therapeutic alliance between you and the patient. The proper environment also allows the pharmacist to focus on providing patient care services rather than attempting to simultaneously perform more traditional pharmacy duties.

Several factors need to be considered when creating the appropriate environment in an ambulatory care practice site. These factors include where the practice is located (e.g., a community pharmacy, a health maintenance organization [HMO], or a physician's office), the physical space where interactions will be conducted, what activities will be conducted in the space (e.g., patient interviews, laboratory testing, or physical assessment), the proximity of this space to other necessary resources (such as clerical support and storage areas), and the types of patients seen in the practice (e.g., diabetic and asthma patients). This unit will address the consideration of each of these factors in various practice settings.

Unit Objectives

After you successfully complete this unit, you will be able to:
- describe important considerations in creating a care office,
- describe how the practice setting may affect the design of the care office, and
- determine additional care office requirements based on the type of practice setting.

Unit Organization

This unit begins with a discussion of factors important to consider when creating a care unit in a retail or community setting. This setting is then compared with a care unit in an HMO, a clinic, or a physician's office. Additional considerations for specialized services are then discussed. The unit concludes with floor planning, and several examples are presented.

Considerations Based on Individual Setting

Retail/Community Pharmacy Setting

Physical Space
The following considerations are critical to the design of a patient care area in a retail/community pharmacy setting, which will be referred to as the *care office*.

Adequate Space
A comfortable environment is important. The care office should be large enough for three to four people to maneuver, sit, and talk comfortably. It is not unusual for a caregiver or significant other to accompany a patient during an appointment. Other health care practitioners or students may also be present. Adequate space for comfortably conducting all the activities to be performed in the care office is crucial. These activities may include patient interviews, physical assessment, and laboratory testing. For example, during a visit, blood pressure readings may need to be taken from a patient's right and left arms. Insufficient space will severely restrict the maneuvering necessary to perform this activity. The care office should be large enough to accommodate the storage and easy access and retrieval of support materials, such as patient records, patient education materials, resource books, and office supplies. These items do not have to be stored in the care office but must be conveniently accessible. Counter or desktop space needs to be adequate for documentation activities (either manual or computer-based) and physical assessment equipment and procedures.

Laboratory testing may or may not be done in the community pharmacy setting. If laboratory testing is done, counter or desk space should be adequate for holding the laboratory instruments and conducting the laboratory procedures. Storage space will be needed for the associated laboratory supplies and the equipment needed for universal precautions (discussed in unit 3).

The care office needs to be accessible for patients with disabilities. There needs to be a doorway wide enough for a wheelchair or walker and adequate space for the patient in a wheelchair to turn around in the office.

Glass Doors and Windows

Consider using glass doors and windows to allow people in the pharmacy to see what is taking place inside the care office. An open or see-through office protects both patients and pharmacists from claims of misconduct. Glass doors and windows also reduce patients' apprehension about this new type of practice by allowing them to view the activities of the pharmacist care office before participating. The new setting prompts questions from potential clients, providing an opportunity to market the program and enroll new patients. With this physical space, you are making a statement that you are committed to the provision of a service. Be aware that some patients and some situations may demand a totally private environment. For example, a patient may be uncomfortable learning to use an inhaler in the view of others. For this reason, consider having blinds to create privacy when needed.

Privacy

The care office should have adequate sound barriers so conversations held in the office are not heard in other areas of the facility. The care office or at least the filing cabinet where patient records are stored must be lockable to maintain patient confidentiality of information. Only personnel working with the patients should have access to the patient records. More on the issue of patient confidentiality is discussed in unit 10, Legal Issues.

Regulations

If any laboratory testing or blood exposure will occur, Occupational Safety and Health Administration (OSHA) regulations must be considered in designing and locating the care office (discussed in unit 3). These regulations require that laboratory activities be conducted near a sink. It may not be practical to have a sink installed in the care office, but one must be nearby and conveniently accessible. If the sink is not in the care office, the person conducting the tests must be able to move to the sink without touching anything, to avoid contaminating any surfaces. For example, doors located between the testing area and the sink must swing open or be able to be pushed open with your body.

Furnishings

A desk and chairs for yourself, the patient, and a possible third party (such as a caregiver) should be arranged in a manner that facilitates communication and allows the performance of necessary monitoring functions. A desk placed between you and the patient may create an intimidating atmosphere and detract from communication. However, this type of arrangement improves eye contact with the patient when a computer is used for documentation purposes during the interview. If the desk is placed between you and the patient, it should be as narrow as possible, to minimize the distance between both parties. A rolling chair for yourself allows you to move easily around the desk if needed to perform monitoring functions. Consider having stationary chairs for the patient and caregiver if you will be seeing patients with limited mobility, such as elderly, blind, or disabled patients. These patients may risk a fall when attempting to sit down in a rolling chair. A list of suggested furnishings and supplies is given in **Table 1**.

Communications

A separate telephone line and answering machine in the care office allows patients to leave messages when no one is available to take their calls without adding to the telephone call volume in the dispensing area. The answering machine decreases interruptions of patient interviews. If you do not choose this option and have patients call the primary pharmacy number, you should establish a policy to ensure that their calls are recorded and passed along to the appropriate person. In any event, tell patients how to reach you in an emergency.

Accessibility

The care office should have convenient access to the pharmacy dispensing area. This convenience facilitates access to dispensing and patient profile information not available in the care office, sharing of reference and resource materials, and coordination of activities between the areas. The care office should also be close to the clerical workers that handle billing or scheduling of appointments. Storage areas for support materials that cannot be kept in the care office should also be convenient, to minimize time spent away from the patient during an interview. If your support materials are stored outside the care office, prepare for each patient visit by locating and gathering all anticipated materials at the point of care.

If possible, the care office should have two doors: one door providing access to the dispensing area, and the other providing outside access for patients. Patients should not have to walk through the main work area of the pharmacy to enter the care office.

Table 1. Suggested Equipment, Furnishings, and Supplies for Care Office

Office Equipment, Furnishings, and Supplies

Business cards
Appointment book or software program
Appointment reminder cards
File cabinet for patient education materials
File cabinet for patient records
Bookcase
Desk
Computer/printer/surge protector (if needed)
Desk chair
Two additional office chairs
Phone
Answering machine
Supplies for patient records
    manila folders
    two-hole punch
    folder labels
Supporting forms
    consent forms
    medical history forms
    care plan forms
    documentation forms
Patient education materials
Reference books

Physical Assessment Supplies

Stethoscope
Professional weight scales
Tape measure or other means to measure height
Mercury sphygmomanometer (desktop model)
Blood pressure cuffs
    standard adult size
    adult large
    pediatric
    thigh

Waiting Area

Outside the care office, there should be an area where patients can sit comfortably while waiting to see you. This area may be a good place to display education materials for patients and advertise your services.

HMO/Clinic/Physician's Office Setting

In other settings, such as HMOs, clinics, or physician's offices, pharmacists may not have as much control over the space available for seeing patients. You are more likely to work in an examination room used primarily by other providers. If this is the case, you will have to adapt the recommendations presented above to your current circumstances. Make sure you have at least a desk to work from and chairs for yourself and the patient. You do not want the patient to have to sit on an examination table during the interaction.

In these settings, sometimes a permanent space to see patients is not assigned. The pharmacist is therefore much more mobile and must gather materials together each day in anticipation of that day's appointments and devise ways to transport them. In addition, sometimes a private room will not be available in these settings, and patients must be seen in a makeshift space, such as a hallway or a semipartitioned area of a waiting room or office. Remember to maximize privacy no matter what the circumstances.

In the HMO, clinic, or physician's office setting, if you have the opportunity to design your office space, the majority of the recommendations about use of space are the same as those for the community pharmacy setting. You do not need two doors into the office, a window, or glass door. An ideal location would be one within the normal flow of patient care activities, so your services are recognized by the other health care professionals working in the area. This proximity allows them to see what you do with patients and seek your advice or refer patients to you. Being in the normal flow of activities also allows you to have access to the other health care professionals for assistance when needed. It would be preferable to be located near frequently used resources, such as clerical support and resource books.

In these settings, you may be conducting laboratory testing during patient visits. Whether you do will depend on access to laboratory facilities, turnaround time for results, and financial and regulatory considerations within the setting. For example, an HMO may allow you to do prothrombin time testing on patients in an anticoagulation clinic because the laboratory the patient would have to use is located several miles away. Alternately, you may not be able to conduct hemoglobin A_{1c} testing on diabetic patients because the clinic laboratory can provide the service at a significantly lower cost. If you are performing laboratory testing within your practice setting, the laboratory considerations discussed under the community pharmacy setting and in unit 3 must be followed.

Considerations Based on Practice Type

In addition to the general list of items in **Table 1**, the laboratory equipment and physical assessment supplies necessary for a practice site will depend on the types of patients seen. For example, in an asthma management practice, you would need peak flow meters and placebo inhalers. In a hyperlipidemia management practice, you would need a lipid analyzer if you were doing the laboratory testing. For each specialized practice site, you will need disease- and medication-specific patient education materials. **Table 2** provides a list of the additional items needed by specialized practice sites.

In addition, the extent of a practice will dictate facility design and equipment and supply needs. For example, a practice in which patients are interviewed and educated, and in which medication recommendations are made without any physical assessment or laboratory monitoring, would need less space and significantly less equipment. Remember that privacy for the interaction is still an essential element. A general ambulatory care practice that sees patients with many different conditions and that performs physical assessment and laboratory monitoring

Table 2. Additional Equipment and Supplies for Specialized Practice Sites

Asthma Management

Peak flow meters
   low flow
   adult
Disposable mouthpieces for peak flow meters
Demonstration inhalers
Disease- and medication-specific patient
   education materials

Diabetes Management

Blood glucose meter
Hemoglobin A_{1c} analyzer
Lipid level analyzer
Reagents (for each of the specific analyzers)
Controls (for each of the specific analyzers)
Supplies (for each of the specific analyzers)
Sensory tester for feet (for early detection of
   diabetic neuropathy)
Disease- and medication-specific patient
   education materials

Hypertension Management

Disease- and medication-specific patient
   education materials

Hyperlipidemia Management

Lipid level analyzer
Reagents (for the specific analyzer)
Controls (for the specific analyzer)
Supplies (for the specific analyzer)
Disease- and medication-specific patient
   education materials

Anticoagulation Management

Prothrombin time/INR analyzer
Reagents (for the specific analyzer)
Controls (for the specific analyzer)
Supplies (for the specific analyzer)
Disease- and medication-specific patient
   education materials

will need the maximum amount of space, equipment, and supplies. This is especially true for patient education materials, which would have to cover the full range of possible conditions and medications encountered.

Floor Plans

Some example floor plans are presented at the end of this unit (**Figures 1–3**). These floor plans may not be applicable to all settings, but many of the

design principles are the same for all settings (i.e., maintaining patient privacy).

Summary

No matter where your ambulatory care practice site is, you have to consider the environment in which you interact with patients. This environment needs to be conducive to establishing a pharmacist/patient relationship and providing privacy. The environment also needs to be organized, so you can interact with the patient in an efficient manner.

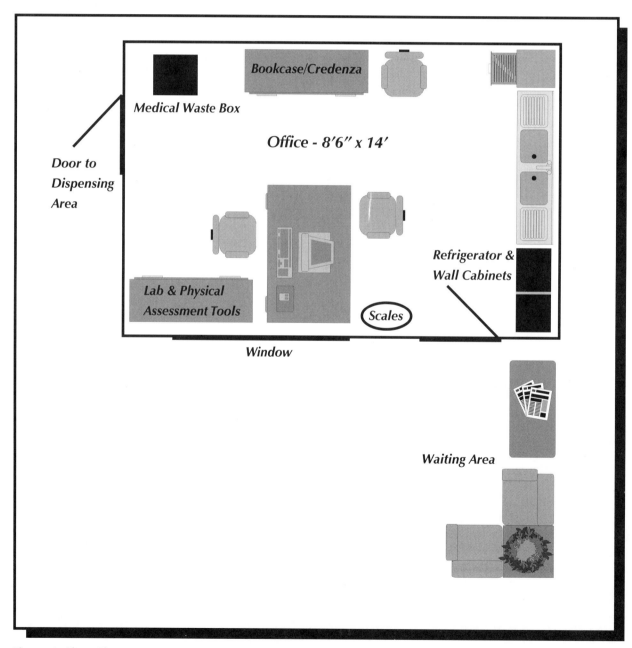

Figure 1. Floor Plan A

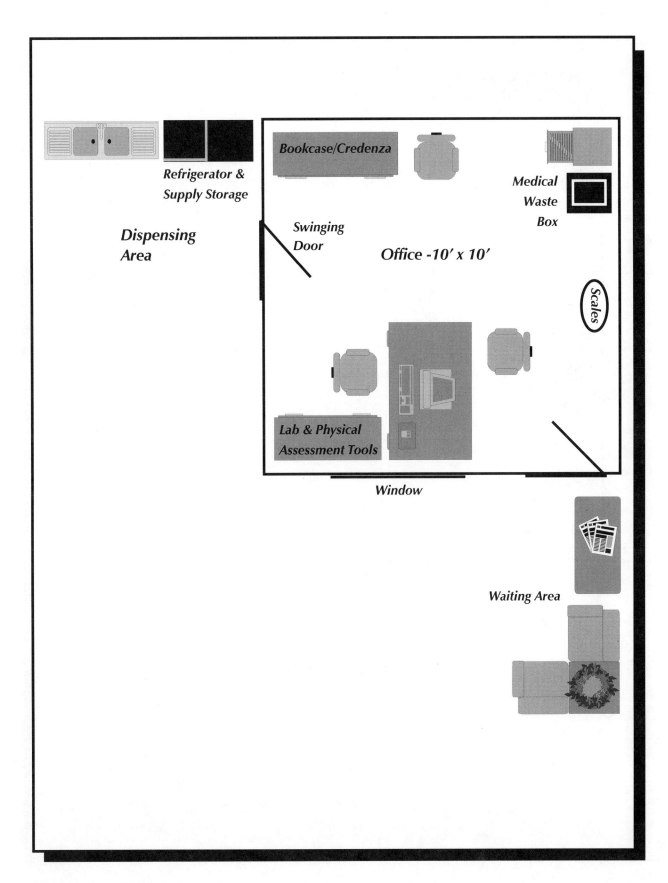

Figure 2. Floor Plan B

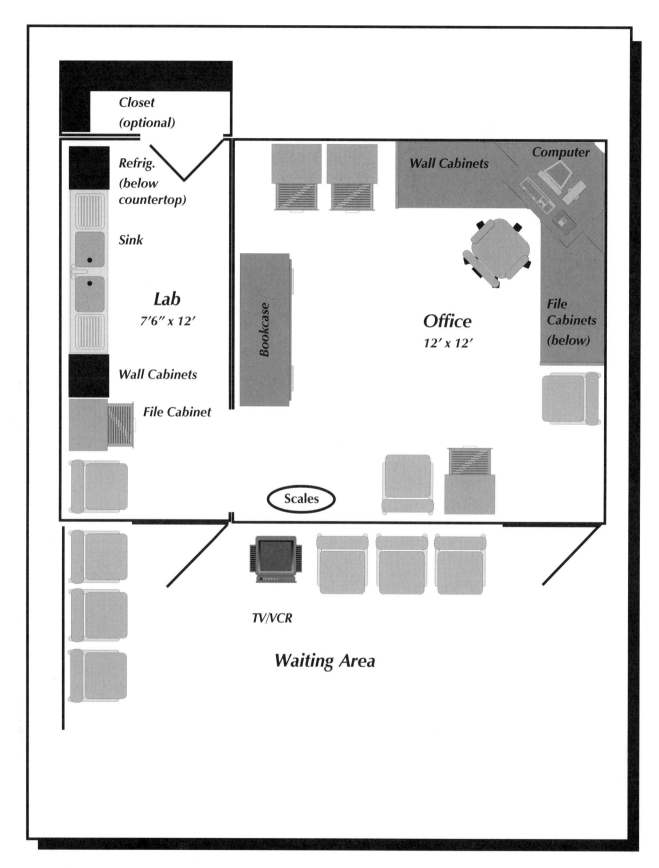

Figure 3. Floor Plan C

Self-Study Questions

Objective

Describe important considerations in creating a care office.

1. Describe factors that need to be considered when allotting space for the care office.

2. Which of the following best describes the use of glass doors and windows in the care office?

   A. It makes for an attractive setting.

   B. It protects care providers and patients from potential litigation.

   C. It allows for increased privacy when counseling.

   D. It allows the pharmacist to view patients in the waiting area.

3. All of the following are designed to protect the privacy of patients *except*:

   A. locked filing cabinets.

   B. sound barriers.

   C. glass doors and windows.

   D. restricted access to patient records.

4. Describe how the location of the care office is important.

Objective

Describe how the practice setting may affect the design of the care office.

5. Which of the following does not describe a possible care office in an HMO, clinic, or physician's office?

   A. The space may be shared with other health care providers.

   B. Its proximity to other patient care activities may increase use of pharmacy services.

   C. The pharmacist may need to transport needed materials, such as educational resources.

   D. The mobile nature of the care office may limit the types of patient care services that the pharmacist can provide.

6. What is a concern common to all practice settings when creating a care office?

Objective

Determine additional care office requirements based on the type of practice setting.

7. Which of the following would most likely be needed in a diabetes management practice?

   A. a lipid analyzer

   B. demonstration inhalers

   C. an INR analyzer

   D. none of the above

Self-Study Answers

1. Factors include the number of people who will normally work in the space (including care providers, patients, and observers), activities to be conducted (including physical assessment, laboratory testing, and documentation), and ability to accommodate equipment used by patients with physical disabilities (e.g., wheelchairs and walkers).

2. B

3. C

4. The location should be convenient to the dispensing and storage areas while not requiring personnel and patients to walk through the main work area. The area should also allow for easy coordination of patient care activities and administrative functions (e.g., billing and scheduling).

5. D

6. Ensuring patient privacy and confidentiality is a primary concern regardless of the practice setting.

7. A

Establishing a Laboratory

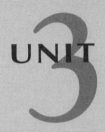

In many ambulatory care settings, the pharmacist may wish to provide laboratory testing in order to:

- facilitate the monitoring and management of drug therapy,
- give patients immediate feedback on progress towards treatment goals, and
- develop a clinical database of laboratory information that is not otherwise readily available.

However limited its scope, pharmacist-conducted laboratory testing in the ambulatory care setting still constitutes operating a laboratory. As such, the laboratory must maintain the same regulatory and quality standards as a full-service laboratory. Depending on its setting, your laboratory may be able to operate under a license already in place (e.g., HMO clinic or doctor's office).

Unit Objectives

After you successfully complete this unit, you will be able to:

- discuss the Clinical Laboratory Improvement Amendments of 1988 (CLIA) and describe how those laws are applied when establishing laboratory services,
- describe Occupational Safety and Health Administration (OSHA) regulations that

must be implemented in the laboratory, and
- discuss laboratory management.

Unit Organization

This unit begins with a review of CLIA and the levels of testing complexity defined by the act. The application of CLIA when establishing a waived and moderate-complexity laboratory is then discussed. Next, OSHA regulations that relate to prevention of bloodborne pathogen or chemical exposure are outlined. Finally, important managerial considerations are described.

CLIA

The Clinical Laboratory Improvement Amendments of 1988 (CLIA) were intended to improve the quality of laboratory services throughout the United States. Since September 1, 1992, CLIA has applied to all laboratories performing tests on human subjects for the purpose of diagnosis, prevention, or treatment of disease. This coverage includes physician office laboratories and pharmacist-conducted testing. CLIA imposes detailed requirements for laboratory personnel, patient test management, quality assurance, quality control, and proficiency testing.

Levels of Complexity

Recognizing that there are different levels of clinical laboratory testing, CLIA bases its required standards on the level of complexity of the tests performed at each laboratory. The classification of a laboratory depends on the highest level of testing it performs. The three defined levels of complexity are:

Waived—Tests in the waived category have been determined to be such simple tests that the risk of an erroneous result is insignificant and, even if performed incorrectly, these tests do not place patients at significant risk of harm. In all cases these are tests designed for patient home use and approved by the Food and Drug Administration (FDA). Waived tests commonly performed by pharmacists are listed in **Table 1**. Laboratories performing waived tests must obtain a Certificate of Waiver and maintain good laboratory practices.

Moderate—Moderate-complexity tests include FDA-approved test methodologies that, if performed according to the manufacturer's instructions, preclude the possibility of life-threatening errors. Laboratories performing moderate-complexity tests must meet requirements for personnel, patient test management, quality assurance, quality control, and proficiency testing to obtain a Certificate of Compliance. Examples of moderate-complexity tests are theophylline levels measured with the Abbott Vision desktop analyzer and serum electrolyte levels such as sodium, potassium, and chloride.

High—High-complexity tests involve extensive manual manipulation, sophisticated technology, or extensive interpretation of test results. The requirements for laboratories performing high-complexity tests are the same as those for moderate-complexity laboratories, with additional requirements in the areas of personnel and quality control. In general, pharmacists do not perform tests of this complexity. An example of a high-complexity test is a complete blood count with differential.

Table 1. Commonly Performed Waived Tests, with Examples of Instruments Used

Blood Glucose

Accu-Chek Easy, Accu-Check Advantage (Boehringer Mannheim)
Glucometer ELITE, Glucometer DEX, Glucometer ENCORE (Bayer)
One Touch Basic, SureStep, One Touch Profile (LifeScan)

Hemoglobin A$_{1c}$

DCA 2000+ (Bayer, also measures urine microalbumin and creatinine, which are not waived)

Fructosamine

Duet Glucose Control System (LXN, also measures glucose)

Cholesterol

Cholestech L-D-X (Cholestech, measures glucose and full lipid profile: total and HDL cholesterol and triglycerides)
CholesTrak (ChemTrak, total cholesterol only)
ChemTrak Accumeter (ChemTrak total cholesterol only)
Accu-Chek Instant Plus (Boehringer Mannheim, total cholesterol only, also measures glucose)

Coagulation

Coagu-Check (Boehringer Mannheim)
Protime Microcoagulation System (International Technidyne Corporation)

CLIA Certification Process

The Health Care Financing Administration (HCFA) is responsible for implementing CLIA, coordinating laboratory certification, and monitoring compliance. Each state has an agency responsible for regulating laboratories and may have requirements that go above and beyond CLIA regulations. You should be aware of the differences between federal and state law and operate the laboratory accordingly. **Table 2** contains a directory of state agencies responsible for laboratory regulation.

Each laboratory must have its own certification and be certified at the highest level of test complexity being performed. For example, even if a community pharmacy is part of a chain, each laboratory site must have its own CLIA certification. In the hospital clinic or HMO setting, however, you may be operating under the license of the main laboratory for the facility.

In general, the following steps are required for CLIA certification:

- Contact the state agency for the state in which the laboratory is located and inform them that you wish to apply for a Certificate of Waiver or a Certificate of Compliance. The state agency will send a CLIA application, HCFA Form 116, and provide other information regarding additional information needed to fulfill state requirements beyond CLIA. A copy of HCFA Form 116 is given in **Appendix A**.
- A waived laboratory will apply for a Certificate of Waiver, and a moderate-complexity laboratory, for a Certificate of Compliance (designated as Certificate on your CLIA application). Complete the application form and return it to the state agency. The owner of the laboratory must sign the application.
- On receiving the application, HCFA will assign the laboratory a CLIA number and mail a CLIA Fee Remittance Coupon to you. Complete and return the coupon, and include the registration certificate user fee. Currently, the biennial fee for a Certificate of Waiver is $100. HCFA has established a fee schedule for moderate-complexity laboratories based on test volume and specialties. Initially (and probably always), the moderate-complexity laboratory will fall into Schedule A (Low Volume, 2,000–10,000 tests annually, with no more than three specialties [e.g., chemistry, hematology,

etc.]). The estimate of your volume is based on the potential number of patients in your practice and the tests performed. Each test is counted for volume, not specimens. For example, a lipid profile (total cholesterol, HDL, and triglycerides) performed on one patient counts as three tests. Test volumes must be updated at least once every 2 years, but sooner if the total exceeds the upper limit. The current biennial fee for Schedule A is $100.

- The laboratory may begin testing after receiving its CLIA number, which generally requires 4–8 weeks. If you do not receive a CLIA number in 8 weeks, call your state or regional office concerning the status of your application.
- The laboratory will receive a registration certificate 6–12 weeks following receipt of fees. This registration certificate is valid for 2 years. Keep this on file in the laboratory at all times.

The remainder of this section will focus on the requirements for establishing moderate-complexity and waived laboratories.

Establishing a Moderate-Complexity Laboratory

As discussed earlier, laboratories performing moderate-complexity tests must meet specific requirements for personnel, patient test management, quality assurance, quality control, and proficiency testing to obtain a Certificate of Compliance.

Personnel

The minimum personnel required for a moderate-complexity laboratory is a laboratory director, a clinical consultant, a technical consultant, and testing personnel. Before applying for a registration certificate for a moderate-complexity laboratory, you must recruit laboratory professionals who meet CLIA personnel requirements.

Laboratory Director

Most pharmacists do not have the educational or technical laboratory experience to meet CLIA personnel requirements for laboratory director of a moderate-complexity laboratory. The position of laboratory director must be filled before submitting the certificate application to CLIA. The laboratory director has responsibility for ensuring that the laboratory meets and maintains CLIA requirements.

Table 2. State Agencies Responsible for Laboratory Regulation

Alabama
Alabama Department of Public Health
L & C Moffit Bldg.
434 Monroe Street
Montgomery, AL 36130-1701
(334) 240-3503

Alaska
Health Facilities Licensure Certification
Department of Health & Social Services
4730 Business Park Blvd.
Suite 18
Anchorage, AK 99503-7137
(907) 561-8081

Arizona
Arizona Dept. of Health Services
Office of Licensing and Certification
Div. of State Laboratory Services
3443 North Central, Suite 810
Phoenix, AZ 85012
(602) 255-3454

Arkansas
Division of Health Facility Services
Arkansas Department of Health
5800 West 10th Street
Little Rock, AR 72205-9912
(501) 661-2201

California
California Department of Health Services
Laboratory Field Services Section
111 Grand Avenue, 9th Floor
Oakland, CA 94612
(510) 873-6327

Colorado
Department of Public Health & Environment
Division of Laboratories
CDH-CLIA Programs
P. O. Box 17123
Denver, CO 80217
(303) 691-4712

Connecticut
Department of Public Health & Addiction
Bureau of Laboratories
150 Washington Street
Hartford, CT 06106
(860) 566-3927

Delaware
Office of Health Facilities
Certification & Licensure
3 Mill Road, Suite 308
Wilmington, DE 19806
(302) 577-6666

District of Columbia
Department of Consumer & Regulatory Affairs
614 H Street NW, Suite 1007
Washington, DC 20001
(202) 727-7200

Florida
State of Florida
Agency for Health Care Administration
2727 Mahan Drive
Tallahassee, FL 32308
(904) 487-2527

Georgia
Georgia Department of Human Resources
Office of Regulatory Services
2 Peachtree Street 21-325
Atlanta, GA 30303-3167
(404) 657-5701

Hawaii
Department of Health
Hospital and Medical Facilities Branch
1270 Queen Emma Street, Suite 1100
Honolulu, HI 96813
(808) 586-4090

Idaho
Laboratory Improvement Section
Bureau of Laboratories
2220 Old Penitentiary Road
Boise, ID 83712-8299
(208) 334-2235

Illinois
Illinois Department of Public Health
Laboratory Regulations Unit
525 W. Jefferson Street, 4th Floor
Springfield, IL 62761
(217) 782-6747

Indiana
Indiana State Department of Health
Division of Acute Care Services
1330 W. Michigan Street
Box 1964
Indianapolis, IN 46206-1964
(317) 383-6502

Table 2. State Agencies Responsible for Laboratory Regulation (cont.)

Iowa
Division of Health Facilities
Iowa Department of Inspections & Appeals
Lucas State Office Building, 3rd Floor
Des Moines, IA 50319
(515) 281-3765

Kansas
Kansas Department of Health & Environment
Laboratory Certification
Building 740, Forbes Field
Topeka, KS 66620
(913) 296-1638

Kentucky
Division of Licensing & Certification
Office of Inspector General
Department of Human Resources
275 E. Main Street
Frankfort, KY 40602
(502) 564-2800

Louisiana
Department of Health and Hospitals
P. O. Box 3767
Baton Rouge, LA 70804-3767
(504) 342-9324

Maine
Department of Health
Bureau of Medical Services
Division of Licensing & Certification
State House Station #11
Augusta, ME 04330
(207) 624-5402

Maryland
Office of Licensing & Certification Programs
Division of Laboratory Licensure
4201 Patterson Avenue, 4th Floor
Baltimore, MD 21215
(410) 764-4695

Massachusetts
Clinical Laboratory Program
305 South Street, Room 224
Jamaica Plain, MA 02130
(617) 983-6739

Michigan
Michigan Department of Public Health
3500 North Logan
Box 30035
Lansing, MI 48909
(517) 321-6816

Minnesota
Minnesota Department of Health
Survey & Certification Section
393 N. Dunlap Street
Box 64900
St. Paul, MN 55164-0900
(612) 643-2104

Mississippi
Licensure and Certification
Mississippi Department of Public Health
P. O. Box 1700
Jackson, MS 39215-1700
(601) 354-7300

Missouri
CLIA Program
Bureau of Hospital Licensing & Certification
P. O. Box 570
Jefferson City, MO 65102
(314) 751-6318

Montana
Licensure & Certification Bureau, Quality
    Assurance Division
Department of Health & Human Services
CLIA Program
Cogswell Building
Helena, MT 59620
(406) 444-1451

Nebraska
Consumer Safety Section
Division of Environmental Health
State Health Department
P. O. Box 95007
Lincoln, NE 68509-5007
(402) 471-0928

Nevada
Nevada Department of Human Resources
Bureau of Lic. & Cert., Laboratory Section
1550 E. College Parkway
Suite 15B Capitol Complex
Carson City, NV 89710
(702) 687-4475

New Hampshire
Department of Health & Human Services
Health Facilities Administration
6 Hazen Drive
Concord, NH 03301
(603) 271-4832

New Jersey
New Jersey State Department of Health
Clinical Laboratory Improvement Program
CN 360
Trenton, NJ 08625-0360
(609) 530-6172

New Mexico
Health Facility Licensing & Cert. Bureau
Public Health Division, Dept. of Health
525 Camino De Los Marquez, Suite 2
Santa Fe, NM 87501
(505) 827-4200

New York
New York State Department of Health
CLIA Unit, Empire State Plaza
P. O. Box 509
Albany, NY 12201-0509
(518) 485-5352

North Carolina
North Carolina Dept. of Human Services
Division of Facility Services
Certification Secretary
701 Barbour Drive
Raleigh, NC 27626-0530
(919) 733-7461

North Dakota
Department of Health & Consolidated Labs
Health Resources Section, CLIA Program
600 East Boulevard Avenue
Bismarck, ND 58505-0200
(701) 328-2352

Ohio
Ohio Department of Health
Laboratory Certification Branch
246 N. High Street
3rd Floor
Columbus, OH 43266
(614) 644-1845

Oklahoma
Oklahoma State Department of Health
Special Health Services
Medical Facilities
1000 NE 10th Street
Oklahoma City, OK 73117-1299
(405) 271-6576

Oregon
Public Health Laboratories
CLIA Program Coordinator
P. O. Box 275
Portland, OR 97207-0231
(503) 229-5854

Pennsylvania
Pennsylvania Department of Health
Bureau of Laboratories
P. O. Box 500
Exton, PA 19341-0500
(610) 363-8500

Rhode Island
Rhode Island Dept. of Public Health
Div. of Facilities Regulation
3 Capitol Hill
Providence, RI 02908-5097
(401) 277-2566

South Carolina
South Carolina Department of Health &
   Environmental Control
Bureau of Certification
2600 Bull Street
Columbia, SC 29201
(803) 737-7205

South Dakota
Licensure & Certification Program
Division of Public Health
South Dakota Department of Health
CLIA Program, 445 E. Capitol
Pierre, SD 57501-3182
(605) 773-3694

Tennessee
Tennessee State Agency
Health Care Facilities
Tennessee Dept. of Health & Environment
283 Plus Park Blvd.
Nashville, TN 37317-0530
(615) 367-6316

Texas
Health Facility Certification Division
Texas Department of Health
1100 West 49th Street
Austin, TX 78756-3199
(512) 834-6650

Utah
Bureau of Laboratory Improvement
Division of Laboratory Services
Utah Department of Health
CLIA Program, 46 N. Medical Drive
Salt Lake City, UT 84113-1105
(801) 584-8469

Vermont
CLIA Laboratory Program
Vermont Department of Health Laboratory
195 Colchester Avenue
Burlington, VT 05402-1125
(802) 863-7565

Table 2. State Agencies Responsible for Laboratory Regulation (cont.)

Virginia
Virginia Department of Health
Office of Health Facility Regulation
3600 Centre Ste. 216
3600 West Broad Street
Richmond, VA 23230
(804) 367-2104

Washington
Office of Laboratory Quality Assurance
Department of Health
1610 NE 150th Street
Seattle, WA 98155-9701
(206) 361-2806

West Virginia
West Virginia Department of Health
Health Facilities Licensure & Certification
1900 Kanawha Blvd. East
Bldg. 3, Room 550
Charleston, WV 25305
(304) 558-0050

Wisconsin
Wisconsin Department of Health & Social
  Services
Division of Health
Clinical Laboratory Unit
P. O. Box 309
Madison, WI 53701
(608) 266-5753

Wyoming
Wyoming Department of Health
Div. of Preventive Medicine, CLIA Program
2300 Capitol Avenue
Hathaway Bldg., 5th Flr., Room 591
Cheyenne, WY 82002-0710
(307) 777-6057

Minimum qualifications for the laboratory director are:
- a bachelor's degree in a chemical, physical, or biological science or medical technology from an accredited institution,
- at least 2 years of laboratory training or experience, and
- at least 2 years of supervisory laboratory experience.

Physicians also qualify as laboratory directors.

The laboratory director does not have to be a full-time employee, but he or she must be available at any time and assumes full responsibility for the laboratory. The laboratory director may delegate, in writing, all of his or her responsibilities to qualified individuals, eliminating the need to be physically present at the laboratory. However, delegation does not relieve the laboratory director from liability or responsibility. The most crucial aspect of the laboratory director's job is to keep the laboratory CLIA certified. The successful candidate should not only meet the supervisory requirement but should also have a working knowledge of CLIA.

One way to recruit a laboratory director is to place a personnel advertisement in the local paper. The advertisement should seek an individual with the minimal experience described above plus an additional requirement for a working knowledge of CLIA. Indicate that the directorship is a part-time position. Another recruitment option is to contact likely sources within your community, for example:
- laboratory manager/supervisor at local community hospital,
- physician's office laboratory,
- a local reference laboratory,
- the Yellow Pages listing for laboratory consultants, or
- university hospitals, a local school of medical technology, or the medical laboratory technician program at a local community college (faculty in these programs would have the credentials to meet CLIA standards).

The financial arrangement made with the laboratory director would vary, depending on the qualifications and the salary base in your area. Initially, the laboratory director will spend a significant amount of time establishing the laboratory (approximately 20 hours), but he or she should routinely spend no more than 3 hours per month overseeing the laboratory after it is running.

Technical Consultant

For moderate-complexity testing, the laboratory must employ at least one individual qualified to provide technical consultation. The technical consultant is responsible for the technical and scientific oversight of the laboratory. The laboratory director may function as the technical consultant in a moderate-complexity laboratory.

Clinical Consultant

The clinical consultant provides consultation and medical opinions to the laboratory's clients concerning the diagnosis, treatment, and management of patient care. The clinical consultant must be a doctor of medicine or osteopathy and must possess a license to practice medicine or osteopathy in the state in which the laboratory is located. A copy of the clinical consultant's current medical license must be on file in the laboratory. Candidates for a clinical consultant include:

- a physician on staff at the clinic or hospital where the laboratory is located,
- a local physician with whom an established professional relationship exists, or
- a pathologist at a local community hospital or group practice.

The clinical consultant need not be a full-time employee and does not need to be on site while testing is performed. An appropriate financial arrangement for the clinical consultant may be a fixed rate per consultation required.

Testing Personnel

Before analyzing patient specimens, each individual performing moderate-complexity testing must, at a minimum, have a high school diploma or equivalent and have documentation of training. The laboratory director is responsible for providing and documenting all necessary training. Depending on state requirements, each individual performing moderate-complexity testing may have to obtain licensure in that state. The laboratory director must ensure that all regulatory requirements in your state are fulfilled before tests can be conducted.

Personnel Documentation

Position qualification forms and detailed listings of the responsibilities for each type of employee involved in moderate-complexity testing are available from HCFA. A position qualification form should be completed for each individual employed by the laboratory. These forms, along with copies of diplomas, certifications, licensure, and resumes, must be maintained as documentation necessary for CLIA in personnel records kept in the laboratory. The forms must be updated whenever changes in personnel occur.

Policies and Procedures Manual

The laboratory must have a written policies and procedures manual, also known as a *standard operating procedures* (SOP) manual. The SOP manual is written documentation of all policies and procedures used in the laboratory. Procedures are written in a stepwise manner, permitting qualified personnel to correctly perform a test or procedure. An example of an SOP for using the Accu-Chek Advantage monitor is given in **Appendix B**.

Patient Test Management

The laboratory must have a patient test management plan that includes written procedures for specimen collection and handling as well as test requisitions and reports. An example procedure for specimen collection and handling is given in **Appendix C**. A test requisition documents the test ordered by the authorized person, and the test report provides written documentation of the test result. CLIA defines the authorized person as anyone allowed by law to order laboratory tests. The two functions can be combined as shown in **Appendix D**. The report must include the name and address of the laboratory in addition to patient-specific information. This report must be maintained in the patient's medical record.

Because requirements can vary from state to state, check with your state agency to ensure that your documentation of patient test results adhere to your state's specific requirements.

Quality Assurance

Moderate-complexity laboratories must have in place a program designed to monitor and evaluate the ongoing and overall quality of the entire testing process, including the preanalytic, analytic, and postanalytic phases of testing. The laboratory director or designee must review this quality assurance (QA) program monthly to ensure that the laboratory is maintaining an acceptable level of performance. Appropriate courses of action to remedy a quality control defect must be documented and reviewed as well. The laboratory director must ensure that all components of the QA program are in place and operational. An example QA program is in **Appendix E**. CLIA requires regular, documented review of the entire QA program. Regular review is usually done on a monthly basis. However, more frequent review may be necessary if a problem area is identified. If a problem area is identified, a plan of action to correct the problem must be outlined, documented, instituted, and then monitored for effectiveness.

The following items must be included in the QA program:

- quality control,
- test comparisons,
- communications,
- staff QA review,
- patient test management,
- proficiency testing,
- personnel assessment,
- complaints,
- QA records, and
- correlation between test results and clinical data.

Quality Control

Quality control (QC) is a system to ensure the technical skill of the laboratory and its personnel. An acceptable QC range for each test is provided by the test manufacturer. QC test results that are out of range indicate a deficiency in the testing process. Appropriate action (recalibration, etc.) needs to be taken before conducting tests on patient specimens if an out-of-range QC result is obtained.

CLIA requires that controls be analyzed according to the instructions from the manufacturer of the laboratory instruments. For example, if the procedure manual for an instrument specifies running a high and low set of controls with each new lot of test strips, then you must run controls at these times to satisfy CLIA regulations. QC materials (e.g., control solutions) are available from the manufacturers of instruments used in the laboratory. QC results must be documented for review and to track trends. An example form for tracking QC results is given in **Appendix F.**

Records of instrument maintenance and temperature checks on the refrigerator are also a part of QC. Whenever reagents, calibrators, or controls require refrigeration, refrigerator temperatures must be monitored and recorded daily to prove that these items are being stored at the appropriate temperature. Instrument maintenance forms must be completed whenever any maintenance is performed on the instrument. Sample forms are included in **Appendixes G** and **H.**

Proficiency Testing

Moderate- and high-complexity laboratories are required to enroll in an approved proficiency testing (PT) program for the laboratory tests they conduct. For example, if a laboratory provides lipid profiles only, it would enroll in a PT program for lipid profile testing. The PT program provider would send the enrolled laboratory prepared samples with known concentrations, for each test that the laboratory is enrolled for. The laboratory submits their results to the PT provider, which compiles the results to yield a group mean and a range of acceptable results based on CLIA standards. Each laboratory's results are then compared with the acceptable ranges and are submitted to the state agency responsible for administering CLIA. Laboratories not performing to the level of acceptability established by CLIA will be subject to disciplinary measures (i.e., revocation of certificate). The PT process is important because it gives each laboratory an objective evaluation of its analytic performance.

PT is performed yearly. The number of sets of samples that are required to be analyzed during a year varies, depending on the laboratory test. Some tests require three sets of samples; others require only two.

A list of approved providers is available from the state agencies responsible for administering CLIA. Some examples of approved providers are given in **Table 3.** Each provider has its own fee schedule. The cost is approximately $50–200 per year, depending on the number of analytes tested.

Other Issues

The laboratory director must also ensure that:

- the laboratory is a proper physical environment for testing,
- testing personnel are competent to perform laboratory procedures,
- communication problems are documented and reviewed,
- complaints are documented and reviewed, and
- test results correlate with patient clinical data.

Proper Physical Environment

The following are principles of providing a proper physical environment for the laboratory instrumentation:

- Laboratory instruments requiring electricity should be plugged into a grounded outlet.
- Extension cords should not be used.
- Instruments should be stored and operated at room temperature (68–82°F) and isolated from direct heat or air conditioning sources.
- A refrigerator that can maintain a temperature of 2–8°C will be necessary to store reagents for the instruments, if refrigeration is specified by the manufacturer. The laboratory refrigerator should not be used to store any food, drinks, or items intended for human consumption. A colored biohazard sticker must be placed on the refrigerator if

Table 3. Approved Proficiency Testing Providers

American Association of Bioanalysts
(800) 234-5315

American Association for Clinical Chemistry
(800) 892-1400

American Proficiency Institute
(800) 333-0958

American Thoracic Society
(212) 315-8808

California Thoracic Society
(714) 730-1944

NY Department of Health
(518) 474-8739

NJ Department of Health
(609) 530-6172

Idaho Department of Health
(208) 334-2235

College of American Pathologists
(800) 323-4040

American Society of Internal Medicine
(800) 338-2746

American Academy of Family Physicians
(800) 274-2237

EXCEL Program, CAP
(800) 323-4040

Wisconsin State Laboratory of Hygiene
(800) 462-5261

Accutest
(800) 356-6788

Puerto Rico Department of Health
(809) 764-6945

Ohio Department of Health
(614) 421-1078

biohazardous materials are stored there. Consider using a small, dormitory-size refrigerator for this purpose.

- A special thermometer must be purchased to monitor the daily temperature of the refrigerator. The thermometer must be traceable to the National Institute of Standards and Technology (NIST) to meet CLIA requirements.

- A source of distilled water is necessary to reconstitute certain materials, such as PT samples or control material, if specified by the manufacturer.

Testing Personnel Competence

The director is responsible for ensuring that qualified and trained individuals perform patient tests. Testing personnel should be trained and assessed for competence initially and then yearly. Documentation of initial training and yearly training checks are required for CLIA inspection. Personnel may not perform real patient testing until all training is complete and properly documented. A sample of a personnel training log is found in **Appendix I** at the end of this unit.

Communication Problems

The laboratory must have a written plan for the documentation of communication problems between an authorized person and the laboratory. Instances of communication problems must be followed up and documented for review by the laboratory director. Acceptable documentation is a memo describing the problem, follow-up, resolution, and action to prevent recurrence of a similar problem. These memos must be kept on file in the laboratory.

Complaints

A system to document complaints about laboratory services must be in place. Complaints should only be accepted in writing, making them official. Appropriate follow-up documentation, with resolution, must be kept on file.

Verifying Test Results

Test results must be verified, based on clinical data (i.e., be appropriate for medical condition, gender, or diagnosis). Records must be reviewed and documentation maintained of any occurrence when results do not correlate.

CLIA Inspection

Inspections by state agencies are performed for moderate-complexity laboratories and can occur anytime after the arrival of the registration certificate. After a successful inspection, the moderate-complexity laboratory will be issued a certificate. This certificate is good for 2 years and may be renewed after a biennial inspection. A fee is charged at the time of inspection. Currently, this inspection fee is $300 for test volumes <2,000 and $840 for test volumes between 2,000 and 10,000.

Establishing a Waived Laboratory

Personnel Requirements

There are no specific requirements for personnel performing waived tests. A laboratory performing only waived tests does not need to employ or maintain staff, including a laboratory director, technical consultant, and clinical consultant, which are necessary for moderate-complexity and higher testing. However, it is good laboratory practice to ensure that all individuals performing waived tests have read and understand the manufacturer's operating instructions and can operate the equipment in a competent manner. Although waived laboratories have no requirements for testing personnel, it is recommended that testing personnel in waived laboratories demonstrate competence and maintain a training log in his or her personnel file (**Appendix I** at the end of this unit).

Good Laboratory Practice

Waived laboratories must utilize "good laboratory practice" while performing tests. Good laboratory practice includes:

- providing the proper physical environment,
- following the manufacturer's instructions for use,
- establishing a QC system,
- recording patient results, and
- properly using and storing test reagents and controls.

Proper Physical Environment

A proper physical environment, as discussed earlier, must be maintained.

Manufacturer's Instructions for Use

The manufacturer's instructions for use must be followed when performing testing. This includes the testing procedure, running of controls, instrument maintenance, and troubleshooting problems.

QC System

QC results must be obtained for each instrument used, in accordance with the manufacturer's instructions for use. For example, if you are performing cholesterol testing using the Cholestech L-D-X, the manufacturer recommends that high and low controls be run on the machine whenever a new lot of testing cassettes is started. Control results must be recorded using the same type of forms used for moderate-complexity testing (**Appendix G**).

Recording Results

Patient test results must be recorded. Typically, this is done in the patient's record. Because requirements can vary from state to state, check with your state agency to ensure that your documentation of patient test results adhere to your state's specific requirements.

CLIA Inspection Process

Sites performing only waived tests are not inspected by HCFA.

Proficiency Testing

Proficiency testing (PT) is an optional activity for laboratories performing only waived tests. Waived laboratories may wish to participate in PT to demonstrate the accuracy of their results. PT may be a condition of participation in some reimbursement contracts.

Laboratory Safety

The Occupational Safety and Health Administration (OSHA) regulates workplace safety. For the laboratory, this encompasses prevention of hazards to employees from bloodborne pathogens and chemicals. The pertinent OSHA regulations for laboratory safety are:

- Bloodborne Pathogens Standard (29 CFR 1910.1030), and
- Occupational Exposure to Hazardous Chemicals in the Laboratory (29 CFR 1910.1450).

Laboratory safety regulations apply anytime blood is used in the laboratory testing process, no matter what level of testing is performed by the pharmacist.

Localities may require more stringent requirements than OSHA. Pharmacists setting up laboratories should contact the state or regional agency responsible for regulating occupational safety and health for guidance on laboratory safety regulations for their state. This document is only a summary of the most pertinent requirements.

OSHA conducts unannounced inspections of facilities. Unlike the state agencies that enforce CLIA, OSHA has the authority to shut down the laboratory immediately if a violation is deemed a serious threat to the safety of either patients or employees. Large fines and/or imprisonment are possible in addition to the closing of the laboratory. Safety must be taken seriously by everyone in the laboratory.

Bloodborne Pathogens

Under OSHA regulations, all laboratories must provide extensive training and preventive measures to protect workers from bloodborne pathogens. These regulations outline what employees must be taught about the hazards of working with potentially infectious materials and what precautions must be taken to prevent or minimize exposure.

Bloodborne Pathogens Exposure Control Plan

All laboratories must implement a written Bloodborne Pathogens Exposure Control Plan (BPECP) to limit employee exposure and evaluate exposure incidents. A BPECP should include:

- identification of workers performing routine tasks and procedures in the workplace that involve exposure to blood or other potentially infectious materials;
- explanation of the protective measures used in the laboratory, including hepatitis B vaccination; universal precautions; engineering and work practice controls; personal protective equipment; procedures for cleanup, decontamination, and biohazardous waste removal; how hazards are communicated to employees; and record-keeping; and
- an action plan to be taken when an exposure incident occurs, including follow-up and record-keeping.

The plan must be reviewed and updated at least annually or whenever new tasks and procedures affect occupational exposure. A written copy of the BPECP must be available in the laboratory at all times for employees and inspectors. An example BPECP is included as **Appendix J**. Another example plan is available from the OSHA Web site on the Internet (www.osha.gov). This example plan is written specifically for home care but can be adapted for the ambulatory care setting.

Preventive Measures

Hepatitis B Vaccine

The hepatitis B vaccine series must be offered after initial training and within 10 working days of initial assignment, free of charge, to every employee who is at risk for occupational exposure. An employee may refuse the vaccine, but the employee must then sign a waiver. Employees have the right to request the vaccine, even if previously refused. The vaccine regimen consists of three doses of vaccine (one vaccine at one, three, and six months). At the end of the regimen, the individual does not need to be tested for hepatitis B antibody, but he or she can be tested to ensure that the vaccine was effective. Testing personnel do not need to complete the entire vaccination series before performing patient tests, but they must receive at least the first shot.

Universal Precautions

The single most important measure to control transmission of hepatitis B virus (HBV) and human immunodeficiency virus (HIV) is to treat all human blood and other potentially infectious materials as if they were infectious. The regulations outlined by OSHA to prevent or minimize exposure are referred to as *universal precautions*.

Engineering and Work Practice Controls

Engineering and work practice controls are the primary methods to control the transmission of HBV and HIV. Engineering controls include the isolation or removal of hazards from employees. The applicable engineering control in the pharmacy ambulatory care laboratory are:

- use closable, puncture-resistant, leakproof containers, color-coded red or labeled with a biohazard symbol (sharps containers) for disposal of lancets and other sharp objects;
- cover work surfaces with an absorbent, disposable material, such as paper towels and dispose of and replace the material between patients;
- clean work surfaces with a 10% solution of bleach at the end of the work shift and between patients;
- properly label biohazards with fluorescent labels on all storage containers or disposal equipment, including waste bags and medical waste boxes; and
- dispose of biohazardous waste appropriately.

You should first investigate local or state regulations concerning biohazardous waste disposal, then locate a biohazardous waste disposal company to remove waste from the laboratory. BFI Medical Services is an example of a national medical biohazardous waste removal company. Community hospitals, physician's or dentist's offices, dialysis clinics, or reference laboratories may permit you to piggyback on their biohazardous waste system. The biohazardous waste disposal company will provide red, labeled trash bags and a biohazardous waste box for disposal of nonsharp items and sealed sharps containers. Records of biohazardous waste disposal must be maintained. These records should include who you are contracted with for disposal and any receipts for disposal.

Work practice controls reduce the likelihood of exposure by altering the manner in which a task is performed. Applicable work practice controls include:

- wash hands when gloves are removed and as soon as possible after contact with blood or other potentially infectious materials;
- provide a mechanism for immediate eye irrigation, acceptable by state standards, in the event of an exposure incident;
- discard contaminated sharp objects in sharps containers that are accessible, maintained upright, and not allowed to be overfilled;
- do not eat, drink, smoke, apply cosmetics, or handle contact lenses in areas of potential occupational exposure; and
- do not store food or drink in refrigerators or on shelves where blood or potentially infectious materials are present.

Personal Protective Equipment

In addition to using engineering and work practice controls, appropriate personal protective equipment (PPE) must be used to reduce risk of exposure. Proper use of PPE in the laboratory protects against direct exposure to blood or other potentially infectious materials.

The employer must assess the workplace to determine the hazards that might require the use of PPE. Based on the assessed hazards, employers must select and have affected employees use properly fitted PPE. The employer must provide the suitable PPE at no cost to the employee. Employees need to be trained on when PPE is necessary; what PPE is necessary; how to properly wear and adjust PPE; the limitations of PPE; and the proper care, maintenance, useful life, and disposal of PPE.

Appropriate PPE for the laboratory includes nonpermeable, disposable laboratory coats to wear while collecting or analyzing specimens for body protection and nonpermeable disposable gloves for hand protection. Eye protection (safety glasses) should be worn if there is a risk of splashing of blood or other body fluids. There is almost no risk of splashing with the finger stick laboratory tests usually conducted by pharmacists.

Disposable gloves must be disposed of after a single use, whether they appear contaminated or not. Disposable laboratory coats that have been contaminated with blood or other body fluids must also be discarded. Dispose of both only in a biohazard trash bag. A regular laboratory coat may be used for body protection, but if it becomes contaminated with blood it must be laundered appropriately by the employer. Employees may not launder contaminated PPE at home. Specific information about laundering reusable PPE, such as laboratory coats, can be found in the OSHA publications listed at the end of this unit.

Communicating Hazards to Employees

OSHA requires that employees be educated annually on the BPECP. This education involves reviewing potential hazards and the BPECP. Documentation of this review must be placed in each employee's personnel file. The training program must do the following:

- explain the written BPECP;
- explain the epidemiology and symptoms of bloodborne diseases;
- explain the modes of transmission of bloodborne pathogens;
- describe the methods to control transmission of HBV and HIV;
- explain how to recognize occupational exposure;
- inform workers about the availability of free hepatitis B vaccinations, vaccine efficacy, safety, benefits, and administration;
- explain the emergency procedures for and reporting of exposure incidents;
- inform workers of the postexposure evaluation and follow-up available from health care professionals;
- describe how to select, use, remove, handle, decontaminate, and dispose of personal protective clothing and equipment;
- explain the use of labels, signs, and color coding required by the standard; and
- provide a question-and-answer session on training.

The person conducting the training must be knowledgeable about the subject matter as it relates to the laboratory. A pharmacist can perform the training once he or she is trained and understands all aspects of OSHA regulations and the written BPECP. Training can be accomplished in several ways:

- use qualified staff (e.g., a pharmacist with

training or a trainer from another department);
- hire qualified personnel from local health care facilities, hospitals, or laboratories; or
- use a bloodborne pathogen and OSHA regulations training videotape (such training must still include a question-and-answer session).

Some companies that provide OSHA training materials are listed in **Table 4**.

The training must be given before the employee begins working in an area where he or she may be exposed to bloodborne pathogens. The training must be repeated yearly and documented. An example documentation form for training is included in **Appendix I**.

Chemical Exposure

The laboratory must have a Chemical Hygiene Plan for the handling of any chemicals stored in the laboratory. If only biohazardous reagents are used in the laboratory, the BPECP may be substituted for the Chemical Hygiene Plan.

OSHA Consultation

If you have any questions or problems regarding OSHA standards and/or inspection, OSHA has established special consultation programs, free of charge, to employers who request help identifying and correcting specific hazards, want to improve their safety and health programs, and/or need further assistance in training and education. For more information on consultation programs, contact your state office (**Table 5**).

OSHA Written Materials

OSHA publications can be obtained by downloading from the OSHA Web site (www.osha.gov), ordering a printed copy from the Web site, or writing to the U.S. Department of Labor [U.S. Department of Labor, OSHA/OSHA Publications, P.O. Box 37535, Washington D.C. 20013, (202) 219-4667, fax (202) 219-9266]. Some of the relevant publications are:
- All about OSHA (OSHA 256),
- Occupational Exposure to Bloodborne Pathogens (OSHA 3126),
- Personal Protective Equipment (OSHA 3077),
- OSHA Inspections (OSHA 2098), and
- Employer Rights and Responsibilities and Course of Action Following an OSHA Inspection (OSHA 3000).

Table 4. Examples of Companies Offering Employee Training Materials and/or Personal Protective Equipment for Meeting OSHA Regulations

Training Materials
Channing L. Bete Co., Inc.
200 State Road
South Deerfield, MA 01373-0200
(800) 628-7733
www.channing-bete.com

Training Materials and Safety Equipment
Conney Safety Products
3202 Latham Drive
P.O. Box 441900
Madison, WI 53744-4190
(800) 356-9100
www.conney.com

Safety Equipment
North Safety Products
2000 Plainfield Pike
Cranston, RI 02921
(800) 881-0444

A copy of the OSHA Bloodborne Pathogens Standard, Title 29 of the Code of Federal Regulations, is available through the Government Printing Office (GPO), GPO Order No. 069-001-0040-8, for a $2.00 fee. To order, call the GPO at (202) 512-1800.

This discussion of OSHA regulations is only an introduction to the requirements for preventing and minimizing exposure to bloodborne pathogens. The reader is strongly encouraged to consult the written materials available from OSHA and make use of the OSHA consultation services when setting up a laboratory.

Laboratory Management Issues

To prove you are in compliance with the many regulations governing laboratory testing, an organized system for maintaining documentation of laboratory activities is necessary.

Table 5. OSHA Consultation Directory

Alabama
Safe State Program
University of Alabama
432 Martha Parham West
P.O. Box 870388
Tuscaloosa, Alabama 35487
(205) 348-3033
E-mail: bweems@ua.edu

Alaska
ADOL/OSHA Division of Consultation
3301 Eagle Street
P.O. Box 107022
Anchorage, Alaska 99510
(907) 269-4957
E-mail: timothy_bundy@labor.state.ak.us

Arizona
Consultation and Training
Industrial Commission of Arizona
Division of Occupational Safety & Health
800 West Washington
Phoenix, Arizona 85007
(602) 542-5795
E-mail: henry@n245.osha.gov

Arkansas
OSHA Consultation
Arkansas Department of Labor
10421 West Markham
Little Rock, Arkansas 72205
(501) 682-4522
E-mail: clark@n237.osha.gov

California
CAL/OSHA Consultation Service
Department of Industrial Relations
Room 1260
45 Freemont Street
San Francisco, California 94105
(415) 972-8515
E-mail: DCBare@hq.dir.ca.gov

Colorado
Colorado State University
Occupational Safety and Health Section
115 Environmental Health Building
Fort Collins, Colorado 80523
(970) 491-6151
E-mail: rbuchan@lamar.colostate.edu

Connecticut
Connecticut Department of Labor
Division of Occupational Safety & Health
38 Wolcott Hill Road
Wethersfield, Connecticut 06109
(203) 566-4550
E-mail: steve.wjeeter@ct-ce-wethrsfld.osha.gov

Delaware
Delaware Department of Labor
Division of Industrial Affairs
Occupational Safety and Health
4425 Market Street
Wilmington, Delaware 19802
(302) 761-8219
E-mail: ttrznadel@state.de.us

District of Columbia
DC Department of Employment Services
Office of Occupational Safety and Health
950 Upshur Street, N.W.
Washington, DC 20011
(202) 576-6339
E-mail: jcates@n217.osha.gov

Florida
Florida Dept. of Labor and Employment
  Security
7(c)(1) Onsite Consultation Prog. Div.
  of Safety
2002 St. Augustine Road, Building E, Suite 45
Tallahassee, Florida 32399
(850) 922-8955
E-mail: brett_crecco@safety_fl.org

Georgia
7(c)(1) Onsite Consultation Program
Georgia Institute of Technology
O'Keefe Building, Room 22
Atlanta, Georgia 30332
(404) 894-2643
E-mail: paul.middendorf@gtri.gatech.edu

Hawaii
Consultation & Training Branch
Dept. of Labor and Industrial Relations
830 Punchbowl Street
Honolulu, Hawaii 96813
(808) 586-9100
FAX: (808) 586-9099

Idaho

Boise State University, Dept. of Health Studies
1910 University Drive, ET-338A
Boise, Idaho 83725
(208) 385-3283
E-mail: lstokes@bsu.idbsu.edu

Illinois

Illinois Onsite Consultation
Industrial Service Division
Dept. of Commerce & Community Affairs
State of Illinois Center, Suite 3-400
100 West Randolph Street
Chicago, Illinois 60601
(312) 814-2337
E-mail: sfryzel@commerce.state.il.us

Indiana

Bureau of Safety, Education and Training
Division of Labor, Room W195
402 West Washington
Indianapolis, Indiana 46204
(317) 232-2688
E-mail: jon.mack@nin-ce-indianpls.osha.gov

Iowa

7(c)(1) Consultation Program
Iowa Bureau of Labor
1000 East Grand Avenue
Des Moines, Iowa 50319
(515) 281-5352

Kansas

Kansas 7(c)(1) Consultation
Dept. of Human Resources
512 South West 6th Street
Topeka, Kansas 66603
(913) 296-7476
E-mail: rudy.leutzinger@ks-ce-topeka.gov

Kentucky

Division of Education and Training
Kentucky Labor Cabinet
1047 U.S. Highway 127 South
Frankfort, Kentucky 40601
(502) 564-6895
E-mail: arussell@mail.laboratory.state.ky.gov

Louisiana

7(c)(1) Consultation Program
Louisiana Department of Labor
OWC-OSHA Consultation P.O. Box 94094
Baton Rouge, Louisiana 70804
(504) 342-9601
E-mail: oshacons@eatel.net

Maine

Division of Industrial Safety
Maine Bureau of Labor
State House Station #82
Augusta, Maine 04333
(207) 624-6460
E-mail: david.e.wacker@state.me.us

Maryland

Division of Labor and Industry
312 Marshall Avenue, Room 600
Laurel, Maryland 20707
(410) 880-4970

Massachusetts

The Commonwealth of Massachusetts
Dept. of Labor & Industries
1001 Watertown Street
West Newton, Massachusetts 02165
(617) 727-3982
E-mail: jlamalva@N218.osha.gov

Michigan (Health)

Michigan Dept. of Public Health
Division of Occupational Health
3423 North Martin Luther King Boulevard
Lansing, Michigan 48909
(517) 335-8250
E-mail: john.peck@cis.state.mi.us

Michigan (Safety)

Michigan Dept of Consumer & Industry
    Services
7150 Harris Drive
Lansing, Michigan 48909
(517) 322-1809
E-mail: ayalew.kanno@cis.state.mi.us

Minnesota

Department of Labor and Industry
443 LaFayette Road
Saint Paul, Minnesota 55155
(612) 297-2393
E-mail: james.collins@state.mn.us

Mississippi

Mississippi State University
Center for Safety and Health
2906 North State Street, Suite 201
Jackson, Mississippi 39216
(601) 987-3981
E-mail: kelly@n198.osha.gov

Table 5. OSHA Consultation Directory (cont.)

Missouri
Division of Labor Standards
Onsite Consultation Program
Department of Labor and Industrial Relations
3315 West Truman Boulevard
P.O. Box 449
Jefferson City, Missouri 65109
(573) 751-3403
E-mail: rsimmons@services.state.mo.us

Montana
Dept. of Labor and Industry
Bureau of Safety
P.O. Box 1728
Helena, Montana 59624-1728
(406) 444-6418
E-mail: dfolsom@mt.gov

Nebraska
Division of Safety Labor & Safety Standards
Nebraska Department of Labor
State Office Building, Lower Level
301 Centennial Mall, South
Lincoln, Nebraska 68509-5024
(402) 471-4717
E-mail: amy@n214.osha.gov

Nevada
Division of Preventive Safety
Department of Industrial Relations, Suite 106
2500 West Washington
Las Vegas, Nevada 89106
(702) 486-5016
E-mail: dalton.hooks@nv-ce-lasvegas.osha.gov

New Hampshire
New Hampshire Dept. of Health
Division of Public Health Services
6 Hazen Drive
Concord, New Hampshire 03301-6527
(603) 271-2024
E-mail: jake@nh7cl.mv.com

New Jersey
New Jersey Department of Labor
Division of Public Safety and Occupational
 Safety and Health
225 E. State Street
8th Floor West
P.O. Box 953
Trenton, New Jersey 08625-0953
(609) 292-3923
E-mail: carol.farley@nj-c-trenton.osha.gov

New Mexico
New Mexico Environment Dept
Occupational Health and Safety Bureau
525 Camino de Los Marquez, Suite 3
P.O. Box 26110
Santa Fe, New Mexico 87502
(505) 827-4230
(505) 827-4422 FAX
E-mail: deborah@n023.osha.gov

New York
Division of Safety and Health
State Office Campus
Building 12, Room 130
Albany, New York 12240
(518) 457-1169
E-mail: james.rush@ny-ce-albany.osha.gov

North Carolina
Bureau of Consultative Services
North Carolina Dept. of Labor
319 Chapanoke Road, Suite 105
Raleigh, North Carolina 27603-3432
(919) 662-4644
E-mail: wjoyner@mail.dol.state.nc.us

North Dakota
Division of Environmental Engineering
1200 Missouri Avenue, Room 304
Bismarck, North Dakota 58506-5520
(701) 328-5188
E-mail: ccmail.lhuber@ranch.state.nd.us

Ohio
Bureau of Employment Services
145 S. Front Street
Columbus, Ohio 43216
(614) 644-2246
E-mail: owen@n222.osha.gov

Oklahoma
Oklahoma Department of Labor
OSHA Division
4001 North Lincoln Boulevard
Oklahoma City, Oklahoma 73105-5212
(405) 528-1500
E-mail: leslie@n238.osha.gov

Oregon
Department of Consumer and Business Services
Oregon Occupational Safety & Health Division
350 Winter Street NE, Room 430
Salem, Oregon 97310
(800) 922-2689
E-mail: steve.g.beech@state.or.us *or*
    consult.web@state.or.us

Pennsylvania
Indiana University of Pennsylvania
Safety Sciences Department
205 Uhler Hall
Indiana, Pennsylvania 15705-1087
(724) 357-2561
E-mail: rchriste@grove.iup.edu

Puerto Rico
Occupational Safety and Health Office
Dept. of Labor & Human Resources, 21st Floor
505 Munoz Rivera Avenue
Hato Rey, Puerto Rico 00918
(809) 754-2188

Rhode Island
Rhode Island Department of Health
Division of Occupational Health
3 Capital Hill
Providence, Rhode Island 02908
(401) 277-2438
E-mail: oshacon@ids.net

South Carolina
South Carolina Department of Labor
Licensing and Regulation
3600 Forest Drive
P.O. Box 11329
Columbia, South Carolina 29204
(803) 734-9614
FAX: (803) 734-734-9741
E-mail: scoshaovp@infoave.net

South Dakota
Engineering Extension
Onsite Technical Division
South Dakota State University
Box 510
West Hall
907 Harvey Dunn Street
Brookings, South Dakota 57007
(605) 688-4101
E-mail: froehli1@ce.sdstate.edu

Tennessee
OSHA Consultative Services
Tennessee Department of Labor
710 James Robertson Parkway, 3rd Floor
Nashville, Tennessee 37243-0659
(615) 741-7036
E-mail: mike.maenza@tn-c-nashville.osha.gov

Texas
Workers' Health and Safety Division
Workers' Compensation Commission
Southfield Building
4000 South Interstate Highway 35
Austin, Texas 78704
(512) 440-3854
E-mail: margaret.nugent@mail.capnet.state.tx.us

Utah
Utah Industrial Commission
Consultation Services
160 East 300 South
Salt Lake City, Utah 84114-6650
(801) 530-6901
E-mail: icmain.nandetso@state.ut.us

Vermont
Division of Occupational Safety & Health
Vermont Department of Labor and Industry
National Life Building, Drawer 20
Montpelier, Vermont 05602-3401
(802) 828-2765
E-mail: web@labor.laboratory.state.vt.us

Virginia
Virginia Department of Labor and Industry
Occupational Safety and Health
Training and Consultation
13 South 13th Street
Richmond, Virginia 23219
(804) 786-6359
E-mail: njakubecdoli@sprintmail.com

Washington
Washington Dept. of Labor and Industries
Division of Industrial Safety and Health
P.O. Box 44643
Olympia, Washington 98504
(360) 902-5443
E-mail: jame235@lni.wa.gov

West Virginia
West Virginia Department of Labor
Capitol Complex Building #3
1800 East Washington Street, Room 319
Charleston, West Virginia 25305
(304) 558-7890

Table 5. OSHA Consultation Directory (cont.)

Wisconsin (Health)
Wisconsin Department of Health & Human Services
Section of Occupational Health, Room 112
1414 East Washington Avenue
Madison, Wisconsin 53703
(608) 266-8579

Wisconsin (Safety)
Wisconsin Department of Industry
Labor and Human Relations
Bureau of Safety Inspections
401 Pilot Court, Suite C
Waukesha, Wisconsin 53188
(414) 521-5063
E-mail: L1163@n215.osha.gov

Wyoming
Wyoming Department of Employment
Workers' Safety and Compensation Division
Herschler Building, 2 East
122 West 25th Street
Cheyenne, Wyoming 82002
(307) 777-7786

Source: OSHA Web site. Available at: http//:www.osha.gov/oshdir/consult.html; accessed January 1999.

Laboratory Procedure Manual

A laboratory manual is an easy way to have all your laboratory documents assembled in one place. This manual should contain your quality control logs (controls on each instrument used, refrigerator temperature, and any applicable maintenance logs) and any policies and procedures developed for the laboratory.

Laboratory Filing System

Some documents need to be kept separate from the laboratory manual. These include:

Personnel records—To meet OSHA regulations, all laboratories must maintain documentation of accidental exposure to bloodborne pathogens, pregnancy waiver, and hepatitis B vaccination or waiver. These documents should be maintained in individual personnel files. Any records of training, either for CLIA or OSHA, also need to be maintained in personnel files.

Proficiency testing—If you are participating in proficiency testing, establish files for each type of proficiency testing analysis you are performing (e.g., a separate file for cholesterol, glucose, and hemoglobin A_{1c}). Maintain all documents related to proficiency testing in these files.

Laboratory safety—To meet OSHA standards, all laboratories must maintain documents relating to OSHA, the BPECP, hepatitis B/HIV testing, laboratory accidents, and hazardous waste disposal. A file containing laboratory safety forms, a copy of the BPECP, and OSHA documents should be maintained for easy retrieval during times of inspection.

Laboratory administrative file—All correspondence with HCFA or other health care regulatory bodies in your state should be maintained for reference and inspection.

If you have a moderate-complexity laboratory, you will need to maintain additional files for QA, patient test results, complaints, and communication problems.

Record Storage

All laboratory records must be kept on site for a minimum of 2 years. The storage should be secure and provide for quick and accurate retrieval of patient or laboratory records. Patient test results must be maintained as long as patient medical records are kept.

Other Issues

Test reagents are very costly, and although it may seem harmless to perform a couple of "free" tests, it can be a costly venture. Establish a system to inventory test reagents on a regular basis to reduce waste and misuse. Reagent usage should correspond with the number of patients evaluated and controls analyzed. Maintain an inventory of test reagents and other consumable laboratory supplies as necessary for patient visits.

Table 6 provides a list of equipment and supplies that are necessary for the laboratory. You may wish to assign one person to be responsible for maintaining appropriate stock levels of all test reagents and other consumable supplies.

Summary

Although it may seem cumbersome, establishing a laboratory within an ambulatory care pharmacy practice setting is relatively easy. You must consider and take very seriously federal and state regulations governing licensing of laboratories and laboratory safety. By using the information in this unit supplemented by information from individual state agencies responsible for administering CLIA and OSHA regulations, you will be on your way to establishing a quality laboratory service.

Table 6. Laboratory Supplies and Equipment

Refrigerator (for storing testing materials)
Puncture-proof container (for sharps disposal)
Red biohazard trash can liners
Fluorescent biohazard label for refrigerator
Nonpermeable laboratory coats
Eye protection glasses
Eye wash
Nonpermeable gloves
Lancets
Antibacterial hand soap
Antibacterial hand wipes
Alcohol swabs
Adhesive bandages
Gauze pads
Paper towels
Bleach
Spray bottle

Self-Study Questions

Objective

Discuss the Clinical Laboratory Improvement Amendments of 1988 (CLIA) and describe how those laws are applied when establishing laboratory services.

1. All of the following describe CLIA *except:*

    A. It was designed to improve the quality of laboratory services.

    B. Its requirements supersede state regulations.

    C. It defines qualifications for laboratory personnel.

    D. Waived testing laboratory requirements are less restrictive than those for a moderate-complexity laboratory.

2. Define the levels of test complexity defined by CLIA.

3. Which of the following is classified as a moderate-complexity test?

    A. fructosamine

    B. complete blood count with differential

    C. blood glucose level

    D. serum phosphate level

4. Which of the following is true of qualified personnel for a moderate-complexity laboratory?

    A. The director is often a pharmacist.

    B. The director may also perform the duties of the technical consultant.

    C. Testing personnel must have, at minimum, a college degree in a laboratory science.

    D. At least three testing personnel must be employed by the laboratory.

5. Explain personnel requirements for a waived testing laboratory.

6. A moderate-complexity laboratory must maintain a Standard Operating Procedure (SOP) for which of the following?

    A. test specimen collection

    B. test reporting

    C. instructions for use for equipment

    D. all of the above

7. Which of the following best describes quality control (QC) as regulated by CLIA?

    A. It applies only to moderate-complexity laboratories.

    B. Its purpose is to ensure the proper training of laboratory personnel.

    C. It is designed to identify problems in the testing process.

    D. It eliminates the need to maintain maintenance records for equipment.

8. Describe proficiency testing (PT) and explain its purpose.

Objective

Describe Occupational Safety and Health Administration (OSHA) regulations that must be implemented in the laboratory.

9. OSHA regulations for prevention of bloodborne pathogen exposure include all of the following *except:*

    A. implementation of a bloodborne pathogen exposure control plan.

    B. employee education on precautions to prevent exposure.

    C. use of universal precautions and personal protective equipment.

    D. annual HIV infectivity testing for all employees.

10. Before assuming responsibilities, each employee should be offered:

    A. a hepatitis B vaccination series.

    B. an influenza vaccination.

    C. a pneumococcal vaccination.

    D. a hepatitis A vaccination.

11. Define engineering and work practice controls used to control the transmission of bloodborne pathogens.

12. List three examples of personnel protective equipment.

13. List laboratory records that must be maintained separate from the laboratory manual.

14. Laboratory records must be stored on site:

    A. for 10 years.

    B. for 2 months.

    C. for 2 years.

    D. indefinitely.

Self-Study Answers

1. B

2. Waived tests are tests that have been approved by the FDA for patient home use. The risk of an error from these tests is small and would not likely result in risk of patient harm. Moderate-complexity tests include FDA-approved test methodologies that preclude the possibility of life-threatening errors if performed according to the manufacturer's instructions. High-complexity tests involve extensive manual manipulation, sophisticated technology, or extensive interpretation of test results. Both moderate- and high-complexity tests have more stringent requirements in the areas of personnel and quality control than waived tests.

3. D

4. B

5. CLIA does not specify personnel requirements for a waived testing facility, but the employee's competence should be ensured.

6. D

7. C

8. PT occurs when a laboratory conducts and submits tests on samples prepared by a PT program provider. It provides an objective evaluation of the laboratory's performance by verifying that the test results fall within an acceptable range. PT is required for moderate-complexity laboratories but is optional for facilities conducting waived tests.

9. D

10. A

11. Engineering controls involve the isolation or removal of hazards from the work area. Examples include the availability of biohazard containers and bags and frequent cleaning of work surfaces with a 10% solution of bleach. Work practice controls are processes that reduce the likelihood of exposure. These include proper and frequent hand washing and prohibition of eating or drinking in work areas.

12. Examples of personnel protective equipment include nonpermeable laboratory coats, safety glasses, and disposable gloves.

13. Laboratory records that must be maintained separate from the laboratory manual include personnel records, results of proficiency testing, safety documents, and correspondence with health care regulatory agencies.

14. C

Appendix A.   Health Care Financing Agency (HCFA) Form 116

DEPARTMENT OF HEALTH AND HUMAN SERVICES
HEALTH CARE FINANCING ADMINISTRATION

FORM APPROVED
OMB NO. 0938-0581

CLINICAL LABORATORY APPLICATION
CLINICAL LABORATORY IMPROVEMENT AMENDMENTS OF 1988

Public reporting burden for this collection of information is estimated to vary between 30 minutes to 2 hours per response , including time for reviewing instructions, searching existing data sources, gathering and maintaining data needed, and completing and reviewing the collection of information. Send any comments including suggestions for reducing the burden to the Office of Financial Management, HCFA, P.O. Box 26684, Baltimore, MD 21207; and to the Office of Management and Budget, Paperwork Reduction Project (0938-0581), Washington, D.C. 20503.

I. GENERAL INFORMATION

Please check any preprinted information on this part of the form and make any necessary corrections. Complete the rest of the form according to the directions.

CLIA IDENTIFICATION NUMBER	FEDERAL TAX IDENTIFICATION NUMBER		
LABORATORY NAME	TELEPHONE NO. *(include area code)*		
LABORATORY ADDRESS *(number, street)*	CITY	STATE	ZIP
MAILING ADDRESS *(if different from above)*	CITY	STATE	ZIP

NAME OF DIRECTOR *(please print or type)*

last   first   MI

Indicate changes below as needed.

LABORATORY NAME	TELEPHONE NO. *(include area code)*		
LABORATORY ADDRESS *(number, street)*	CITY	STATE	ZIP
MAILING ADDRESS *(if different from above)*	CITY	STATE	ZIP

NAME OF DIRECTOR *(please print or type)*

last   first   MI

II. APPLICATION IS FOR: *(check one box)*

☐ Certificate   ☐ Renewal of Certificate
☐ **Certificate of Waiver   ☐ Renewal of Certificate of Waiver
☐ Certificate of Accreditation   ☐ Renewal of Certificate of Accreditation

**IF YOU CONDUCT ONLY THE FOLLOWING WAIVED TESTS *(ONE OR MORE),* YOU MAY APPLY FOR A CERTIFICATE OF WAIVER:.

•Dipstick or tablet reagent urinalysis (nonautomated) for:
   -bilirubin   -glucose
   -hemoglobin   -ketone
   -leukocytes   -nitrite
   -protein   -pH
   -specific gravity -urobilinogen
•Fecal occult blood
•Ovulation test-visual color comparison tests for human
  luteinizing hormone

•Urine pregnancy test-visual color comparison tests
•Erythrocyte sedimentation rate (nonautomated)
•Hemoglobin-copper sulfate (nonautomated)
•Blood glucose, by glucose monitoring devices cleared by
  the FDA specifically for home use; and
•Spun microhematocrit

If applying for a **certificate of waiver,** complete all sections of this form except section VIII.

FORM HCFA-116 (8-92)   Page 1 of 4

continued on next page

III. TYPE OF LABORATORY *(check the <u>one</u> most descriptive of facility type)*

___ 01 Ambulatory Surgery Center	___ 08 Home Health Agency	___ 15 Mobile Unit
___ 02 Community Clinic	___ 09 Hospice	___ 16 Pharmacy
___ 03 Comp. Outpatient Rehab. Facility	___ 10 Hospital	___ 17 School/Student Health Service
___ 04 Ancillary Testing Site in Health Care Facility	___ 11 Independent	___ 18 Skilled Nursing Facility/Nursing Facility
	___ 12 Industrial	___ 19 Physician Office
___ 05 End Stage Renal Disease Dialysis Facility	___ 13 Insurance	___ 20 Other Practitioner *(specify)* _____
___ 06 Health Fair	___ 14 Intermediate Care Fac. for Mentally Retarded	___ 21 Tissue Bank/Repositories
___ 07 Health Main. Organization		___ 22 Blood Banks
		___ 23 Other *(specify)* _____

Was this <u>laboratory</u> previously regulated under the Federal Medicare/Medicaid and/or CLIA programs? (Regulations published March 14, 1990 at 55 FR 9538) .... ☐ Yes   ☐ No

IV. HOURS OF ROUTINE OPERATION

List days and hours during which <u>laboratory testing</u> is performed

	SUNDAY	MONDAY	TUESDAY	WEDNESDAY	THURSDAY	FRIDAY	SATURDAY
FROM: AM							
PM							
TO: AM							
PM							

(For multiple sites attach the additional information using the same format)

V. MULTIPLE SITES

Are you applying for one certificate for multiple sites?   ☐ No *If no,* go to next section.

☐ Yes *If yes,* total number of sites_____ and complete appropriate section below.

Identify which of the following exception requirements applies to your laboratory operation.

Is this a non-profit or Federal, State or local government laboratory engaged in limited *(e.g., few types of tests)* public health testing and filing for a single certificate for multiple sites? ......☐ Yes   ☐ No
If yes, list name, address and tests performed for each site below.

Is this a hospital with several laboratories at the same street address and under common direction that is filing for a single certificate for these locations? ....☐ Yes   ☐ No
If yes, list name or department, location within hospital and specialty/subspecialty areas for each site below.

If additional space is needed, check here _____ and attach the additional information using the same format.

NAME AND ADDRESS / LOCATION		TESTS PERFORMED / SPECIALTY / SUBSPECIALTY
Name of laboratory or hospital department		
Address/location (number, street, location if applicable)		
City, State, ZIP	Telephone No. ( )	
Name of laboratory or hospital department		
Address/location (number, street, location if applicable)		
City, State, ZIP	Telephone No. ( )	
Name of laboratory or hospital department		
Address/location (number, street, location if applicable)		
City, State, ZIP	Telephone No. ( )	

continued on next page

VI. ACCREDITATION INFORMATION

Is your laboratory presently accredited by any private nonprofit organization ....☐ Yes   ☐ No

Accredited by:

If yes, check all that apply:

☐ JCAHO   ☐ COLA
☐ AOA   ☐ ASC
☐ AABB   ☐ ASHI
☐ CAP   ☐ Other *(specify)* _____

VII. WAIVED TESTING

Indicate total annual test volume for all waived tests performed. _____

VIII. NONWAIVED TESTING

If you perform testing other than or in addition to waived tests, complete the information below. If applying for one certificate for multiple sites, include information for all sites.

Place a check (√) in the box preceding each specialty/subspecialty in which the laboratory performs testing. Enter the test volume for the previous calendar year for each specialty. If you are a new laboratory or have added new specialties/subspecialties, for test volume, enter your estimated annual test volume. Do not include testing not subject to CLIA, waived tests, or tests run for quality control, quality assurance or proficiency testing when estimating total volume. Each profile, panel or group of tests usually performed simultaneously is counted as the total number of separate tests or procedures of which it is comprised. Calculations such as A/G ratio, MCH, MCHC and T_7 are an exception and should not be included in the total count. Examples: A chemistry profile consisting of 18 separate procedures is counted as 18 separate procedures. In the same manner, a CBC is counted as each individual measured (not calculated) analyte and as one test for the differential. For microbiology, susceptability testing is counted as one test per group of antiobiotics used to determine sensitivity for one organism.

If applying for certificate of accreditation, indicate name of current accrediting body beside applicable specialty/subspecialty.

SPECIALTY / SUBSPECIALTY	ACCREDITED PROGRAM	ANNUAL TEST VOLUME	SPECIALTY / SUBSPECIALTY	ACCREDITED PROGRAM	ANNUAL TEST VOLUME
☐ **Histocompatibility**		_____	☐ **Hematology**		_____
☐ Transplant	_____		☐ **Immunohematology**		_____
☐ Non-transplant	_____		☐ ABO Group & Rh Group	_____	
☐ **Microbiology**		_____	☐ Antibody Detection (transfusion)	_____	
☐ Bacteriology	_____				
☐ Mycobacteriology	_____		☐ Antibody Detection (nontransfusion)	_____	
☐ Mycology	_____				
☐ Parasitology	_____		☐ Antibody Identification	_____	
☐ Virology	_____		☐ Compatibility Testing	_____	
☐ Other	_____				
☐ **Diagnostic Immunology**		_____	☐ Other	_____	
☐ Syphilis Serology	_____		☐ **Pathology**		_____
☐ General Immunology	_____		☐ Histopathology		
			☐ Oral Pathology		
☐ **Chemistry**		_____	☐ Cytology		_____
☐ Routine	_____				
☐ Urinalysis	_____		☐ **Radiobioassay**		_____
☐ Endocrinology	_____				
☐ Toxicology	_____		☐ **Clinical Cytogenetics**		_____
☐ Other	_____		**TOTAL ANNUAL TEST VOLUME**		

continued on next page

IX. TYPE OF CONTROL	X. TYPE OF OWNERSHIP
Enter the appropriate two digit code from the list below _____ ____ (enter only one code)	Enter the appropriate two digit code from the list below _____ ____ (enter only one code)

IX. TYPE OF CONTROL

Voluntary Nonprofit
01 Religious Affiliation
02 Private
03 Other

For Profit
04 Proprietary

Government
05 City
06 County
07 State
08 Federal
09 Other Government

X. TYPE OF OWNERSHIP

01 Sole Proprietorship
02 Partnership
03 Corporation
04 Other (specify)

_____

XI. DIRECTOR AFFILIATION WITH OTHER LABORATORIES

If the primary director of this laboratory serves as primary director for laboratories that are separately certified, please complete the following:

NAME OF LABORATORY	ADDRESS	CLIA IDENTIFICATION NUMBER

XII. INDIVIDUALS INVOLVED IN LABORATORY TESTING

Indicate the total number of individuals involved in laboratory testing (directing, supervising, consulting or testing). Do not include individuals who only collect specimens or perform clerical duties. For nonwaived testing, only count an individual one time, at the highest laboratory position in which they function. (Example Pathologist serves as director, technical supervisor and general supervisor. This individual would only be counted once (under director)).

A. Waived TOTAL
No. of Individuals _____

B. Nonwaived TOTAL No. of Individuals _____
Director _____   Technical supervisor _____
Clinical consultant _____   General supervisor _____
Technical consultant _____   Testing personnel _____

ATTENTION: READ THE FOLLOWING CAREFULLY BEFORE SIGNING APPLICATION

ANY PERSON WHO INTENTIONALLY VIOLATES ANY REQUIREMENT OF SECTION 353 OF THE PUBLIC HEALTH SERVICE ACT AS AMENDED OR ANY REGULATION PROMULGATED THEREUNDER SHALL BE IMPRISONED FOR NOT MORE THAN ONE YEAR OR FINED UNDER TITLE 18, UNITED STATES CODE OR BOTH, EXCEPT THAT IF THE CONVICTION IS FOR A SECOND OR SUBSEQUENT VIOLATION OF SUCH A REQUIREMENT SUCH PERSON SHALL BE IMPRISONED FOR NOT MORE THAN 3 YEARS OR FINED IN ACCORDANCE WITH TITLE 18, UNITED STATES CODE OR BOTH.

CONSENT: THE APPLICANT HEREBY AGREES THAT SUCH LABORATORY IDENTIFIED HEREIN WILL BE OPERATED IN ACCORDANCE WITH APPLICABLE STANDARDS FOUND NECESSARY BY THE SECRETARY OF HEALTH AND HUMAN SERVICES TO CARRY OUT THE PURPOSES OF SECTION 353 OF THE PUBLIC HEALTH SERVICE ACT AS AMENDED. THE APPLICANT FURTHER AGREES TO PERMIT THE SECRETARY, OR ANY FEDERAL OFFICER OR EMPLOYEE DULY DESIGNATED BY THE SECRETARY, TO INSPECT THE LABORATORY AND ITS OPERATIONS AND PERTINENT RECORDS AT ANY REASONABLE TIME.

SIGNATURE OF OWNER/AUTHORIZED REPRESENTATIVE OF LABORATORY(sign in ink)   DATE

last   first   MI

APPENDIX B. SAMPLE STANDARD OPERATING PROCEDURE (SOP)

Whole Blood Glucose Testing Using the Accu-Chek Advantage Monitor

Prepared by	Date Adopted	Supersedes Procedure #

Review Date	Revision Date	Signature

Distributed to	# of Copies	Distributed to	# of Copies

Principle:

The Accu-Chek Advantage Monitor is a waived test under CLIA 1988. Therefore a SOP is not mandatory. CLIA does require that good laboratory procedures be followed while performing the testing. Thoroughly read and understand the current package inserts and instructions that come with the Advantage Monitor and/or the Reagent Strips. Follow all instructions as written and do not deviate from the instructions provided by the manufacturer. Record the results of the Quality Control tests for reference in the future.

Specimen:

The specimen used in the PCL will be collected via finger stick method, see *Collection of Capillary Blood Specimen* SOP.

Equipment & Materials:

Minimal equipment is needed for this test.

Equipment: Accu-Chek Advantage Monitor

Materials: Reagent Strips for glugose testing.

Preparation: Reagent strips are ready to use.

Storage Requirements: Reagent strips are stored at room temperature.

continued on next page

Calibration:

No calibration is required.

Quality Control:

Two (2) quality control specimens must be run with each new vial of reagent strips. Follow package inserts for instructions.

Procedure—Stepwise:

Follow manufacturer's instructions for performing test.

Calculations:

No calculations are necessary for this test.

Reporting Results:

Patient results are recorded in the patient's electronic medical record or on a *Test Requisition and Report* form.

Reportable Range: 20–600 mg/dL.

Reference Ranges: Normal Range: 70–110 mg/dL for fasting adults. One to two hours after a meal, normal glucose levels may be 110–180 mg/dL.

Procedures for Abnormal Results: Abnormal Results: <60 mg/dL or >240 mg/dL. Repeat the test if an abnormal result is determined. If the second test is still abnormal and the clinical signs and symptoms do not match the results **the patient's physician should be notified.**

Reporting Format: Patient results will be reported as displayed by the Advantage Monitor. No rounding is to be performed.

Procedure Notes:

Consult manufacturer's instructions for further information.

Limitations of the Procedure:

If test results are not consistent with clinical symptoms, repeat test to confirm. Consult manufacturer's instructions for further information.

References:

1.   Accu-Chek Advantage Monitor Operating Instructions.

APPENDIX C.   EXAMPLE SOP FOR SPECIMEN COLLECTION AND HANDLING

Specimen Collection and Handling

Prepared by	Date Adopted	Supersedes Procedure #	

Review Date	Revision Date	Signature	

Distributed to	# of Copies	Distributed to	# of Copies

Principle:

Proper collection and handling of whole blood specimens is necessary to ensure reliable test results. The initial steps in the procedure are the same for all tests. Specific requirements for each test can be found by referring to the operation manual for each instrument. (You can add these requirements for instruments you will be using.)

Specimen:

The specimen used in the laboratory will be collected via finger stick method. Specimens should be tested within the time limits specified for each instrument. (You can add these specifications for instruments you will be using.)

Equipment and Materials:

Minimal materials are needed.

Materials: Absorbent, nonpermeable cover for work surface   Lancet device for puncturing skin
               Alcohol swabs   Collection device appropriate for test
               Latex gloves   Biohazardous waste container
               Gauze pads   Bandages

continued on next page

Procedure—Stepwise:

Obtaining a proper finger puncture

Choose a site free of cuts and abrasions on one of the four fingers (not the thumb). It is often helpful to ask the patient which finger she/he would like punctured.

Warming the skin can significantly increase the blood flow. Use a warm compress to cover the site for several minutes. Alternatively, gently rub the site to warm it.

Clean the site with an alcohol swab. Do not use povidone iodine. Allow the alcohol to air dry or dry thoroughly with a sterile gauze. Residual alcohol causes hemolysis as well as a burning sensation for the patient.

Puncture the skin to a depth of about 2 mm, enough for adequate blood flow.

Wipe away the first drop of blood with a gauze pad because it may contain excess tissue fluid. Collect blood sample using appropriate device for test (you can specify based on the tests you will be doing). Do not squeeze or milk the finger. This may cause hemolysis or contaminate the sample with tissue fluid.

After blood collection is completed, apply sterile gauze to the puncture site and apply gentle pressure until the bleeding stops. Provide a bandage if the patient desires one.

Discard used materials into the appropriate labeled biohazardous waste container.

References:

(Reference the operating manuals for the instruments you will be using.)

APPENDIX D. TEST REQUISITION AND REPORT

LABORATORY NAME
Address

PATIENT TEST REQUISITION AND REPORT

Patient Name:_____   ID # :_____

Address:_____   Telephone:_____

Date/Time Drawn:_____   Initials:_____

Date/Time Completed:_____   Initials:_____

Health Care Provider:_____   Address:_____

TEST	RESULT	NORMALS	COMMENT
glucose	_____	*76–115 mg/dL	_____
total cholesterol	_____	<200 mg/dL	_____
triglycerides	_____	<250 mg/dL	_____
HDL	_____	≥35 mg/dL	_____
calculated LDL	_____	<130 mg/dL	_____
glycosylated hemoglobin	_____	<7 mg%	_____

* Normal glucose for a fasting adult.

Enter "TNP" if the test was not performed.

Place in the patient's file.

APPENDIX E. EXAMPLE QA PROGRAM

Quality Assurance Program

This laboratory has established the following goals for our Quality Assurance Program. We intend to:

- Evaluate the effectiveness of our written policies and procedures.
- Identify problems in our laboratory and apply corrective action.
- Assure that accurate and reliable test results are obtained and reported to our physicians in a timely manner.
- Assure that laboratory personnel are adequately trained and that their performance is periodically evaluated.
- Revise our laboratory policies and procedures whenever necessary.

Each month, one of the following systems in our laboratory will be evaluated to be sure it meets our quality goals. If a problem is identified, we will design and implement a solution that is approved by the laboratory director. To determine if our plan has worked, we will reevaluate the system in 3 months. We will keep written records of our reviews, findings, and actions.

Patient Test Management

We will evaluate:

- The procedures for patient preparation and specimen collection, labeling, preservation, and transportation.
- The laboratory test requisition requirements.
- The criteria used for specimen rejection.
- The test reporting method for completeness, usefulness and accuracy of the information needed to interpret and use the report.
- The timely reporting of test results based on testing priorities such as stat and routine.

Quality Control and Instrumentation

We will evaluate our quality control program for calibration and control data for each test method used in the lab and determine:

- If calibrators and controls are run according to written policies and procedures.

- If personnel have taken appropriate corrective action when calibration or control values are out of the acceptable range.
- The effect on patient test results when controls or calibrators have been out of the acceptable range and if this caused errors on test reports.

We will evaluate our laboratory instrument use to determine if laboratory staff:

- Follow manufacturer's directions in the operation of the instrument, and
- Follow manufacturer's recommendations for instrument maintenance.

This information will be recorded and kept with our quality assurance records.

Proficiency Testing

We will evaluate the results of our proficiency testing (PT) with the laboratory director within one week of their return from the PT program. We will carefully evaluate any unacceptable, unsatisfactory, or unsuccessful proficiency testing result in an effort to identify the cause of failure. If a cause is found, we will take necessary corrective action and reevaluate the PT results after the next PT challenge. This information will be recorded and kept with our quality assurance records.

Comparison of Test Results

Our laboratory will verify the accuracy of backup instruments or any tests that are not enrolled in a proficiency testing program. We will do so by running at least two split specimens (a specimen that is divided into two parts after collection — the laboratory analyzes one portion and the other is sent to a reference laboratory for analysis) and comparing our results with those of the reference laboratory. Twice a year we will perform this verification on the following instruments, backup methods for tests for which are not enrolled in PT:

INSTRUMENT   ANALYTE

We will establish how many split specimens will be run for each analyte and what we consider an acceptable variation between our result and the

continued on next page

reference laboratory's result (e.g., +/–5%, +/–7.5%, +/–0.6 mEq, etc.). If the results vary more than the acceptable range, staff should determine the possible cause and take action if the cause is within the laboratory. This information will be recorded and kept with our quality assurance records.

Relationship of Patient Information to Patient Results

We will periodically review test reports for consistency of the report with patient information available to the laboratory, including:

- patient age,
- patient gender,
- patient diagnosis or pertinent clinical data,
- distribution of patient test results, and
- the relationship of the patient test results to other test parameters.

Personnel Assessment

To assure employee competence, the pharmacist or laboratory director will annually review the performance of each employee working in the laboratory. The written result of the review will be filed in the individual's personnel file. Opportunities will be made available to laboratory personnel for continuing education and noted in the record at the time of this review.

Communication

We consider effective communication vital to the operation of this laboratory. Every significant breakdown in communication will be recorded and reviewed by the director. Any corrective actions taken to prevent further communication problems will be recorded and reevaluated for effectiveness in six months as part of our quality assurance program. This information will be recorded and kept with our quality assurance records.

Laboratory Errors

We will evaluate all errors made by the laboratory and determine if changes must be made in our policy and procedure to prevent similar errors in the future. As part of this process, we will evaluate the cause of the error, who was notified of the error, whether the physician received a corrected report, and when the corrected report was sent. This information will be recorded on the "Laboratory Errors" form and kept with our quality assurance records.

Complaints

Any complaints about our laboratory, whether from physicians, patients, or staff are taken seriously and will be evaluated promptly. Any actions taken to correct the underlying cause of the complaint will be reviewed by the laboratory director. This information will be recorded and kept with our quality assurance records.

Quality Assurance Review

Our laboratory uses this quality assurance program to improve the laboratory services we provide to our physicians and patients. We will perform a quality review at least monthly and review the results with the laboratory director or technical consultant for their approval. Changes in our policy or procedures resulting from this quality review will be made known to the entire laboratory staff. The laboratory director or consultant will initial and date our written reviews and actions.

Quality Assurance Records

The record of our quality assurance reviews are filed with this plan and are available for review by the director, consultant, staff, and laboratory surveyors. All records are dated and initialed by the staff performing the review, and by the laboratory director.

APPENDIX F. EXAMPLE QUALITY CONTROL CHART

CONTROL __Low__   MEAN _____   MIN. _____   MAX. _____

Date	1	2	3	4	5	6	7	8	9	10	11	12	13	14	15	16	17	18	19	20	21	22	23	24	25	26	27	28	29	30	31
Tech																															
Value																															
Max																															
X																															
Min																															

CONTROL __High__   MEAN _____   MIN. _____   MAX. _____

Date	1	2	3	4	5	6	7	8	9	10	11	12	13	14	15	16	17	18	19	20	21	22	23	24	25	26	27	28	29	30	31
Tech																															
Value																															
Max																															
X																															
Min																															

Self Chk

DATE   CORRECTIVE ACTION   TECH

REAGENT/NAME LOT # _____   EXP DATE _____

Instructions for Use:

1. Provide the acceptable control values as established by the manufacturer or in departmental policy. Transfer these values to the max/min grid and establish a scale for plotting data.
2. For each analysis performed, indicate the person performing the analysis and the value obtained in the initial and value rows, respectively.
3. Plot the value obtained in the grid using the scale established for the equipment or procedure being analyzed.
4. If the result was obtained from the equipment's self-checking feature, check the appropriate box.
5. Record the lot and expiration date of the reagent used, if any.
6. Explain any corrective action taken. Include date and initials.

Appendix G. Example Instrument Maintenance Log

INSTRUMENT MAINTENANCE LOG

CHOLESTECH L-D-X®

SERIAL NUMBER _____

Date	Initials	Optics Check	Other (describe)

REFRIGERATOR TEMPERATURE LOG

REFRIGERATOR ID _____

ACCEPTABLE RANGE 2–8°C

Date	Initials	Temp.	Actions

APPENDIX I. PERSONNEL TRAINING LOG

PERSONNEL TRAINING LOG

NAME_____

Date	Employee Signature	Trainer's Signature	Training Received (add as needed)
BLOODBORNE PATHOGEN EXPOSURE CONTROL PLAN			
			Bloodborne pathogens standards
			Universal precautions
			Protective equipment
			Accidental exposure procedures
LABORATORY OPERATIONS			
			Finger stick procedure
			Instrument operation & maintenance
			Quality control procedures
			Record-keeping procedures
			Proficiency testing (if applicable)
ANNUAL UPDATES			
			Bloodborne Pathogens Exposure Control Plan
			Laboratory Operations

Original: Facility Copy
Duplicate: Personnel File

BLOODBORNE PATHOGEN EXPOSURE CONTROL PLAN

Principle

Occupational Safety and Health Administration (OSHA) requires that all laboratory employees be trained annually on bloodborne pathogens exposure. This Bloodborne Pathogens Exposure Control Plan (BPECP) provides guidance to minimize and prevent the exposure of employees to microorganisms transmitted through human blood. This BPECP will be reviewed at least annually and updated as necessary.

Exposure Determination

All job categories in which it is reasonable to anticipate that an employee may have skin, eye, mucous membrane, or parenteral contact with blood or other potentially infectious materials (listed below) will be included in this BPECP. Exposure determination is made without regard to the use of personal protective equipment (i.e., employees are considered to be exposed to infectious materials even if they wear personal protective equipment).

Potentially Infectious Materials

Potentially infectious materials include:
- Whole blood
- Control solutions for Cholestech L-D-X System
- [add information for particular instruments you would be using if any of the solutions or reagents are derived from blood]

Employees in job categories listed here are included in the plan:
- Testing personnel

Methods of Compliance

Universal Precautions

All blood or other potentially infectious materials (as described above) shall be handled as if contaminated by a bloodborne pathogen.

Engineering and Work Practice Controls

Whenever feasible, engineering and work practice controls shall be installed and used to eliminate or minimize employee exposure. Where the potential for occupational exposure remains after institution of these controls, personal protective equipment shall also be used. The following engineering controls will be available for use as needed:
- Sharps containers for disposal of needles, lancets, etc.

The above devices will be maintained, inspected, and replaced as needed. Schedule for maintenance and inspection will be:
- Daily: Clean and check for defects or need to replace by user.

Hand Washing and Other General Hygiene Measures

Hand washing is a primary infection control measure to provide protection for employees, patients, and coworkers. Appropriate hand washing must be diligently practiced. Employees shall wash hands thoroughly using soap and water as soon as possible after removing gloves or other personal protective equipment. In areas where a sink is not readily accessible, antiseptic towelettes are available for cleaning hands immediately after the removal of gloves and other protective equipment.

Immediately following a needle stick or other sharp contact with introduction of potentially infectious material, the break or puncture in the skin should first be squeezed to induce bleeding and then flushed with water. When skin areas or mucous membranes come in contact with blood or other potentially infectious materials, the skin shall be washed with soap and water and the mucous membranes shall be flushed with water immediately. Employees must contact their supervisor to report mucous membrane or sharps exposures and receive appropriate follow-up. Sinks are provided in each work area where risk of occupational exposure exists. Employees are to request replacement of antiseptic soap and paper towels immediately to housekeeping.

Eating, drinking, smoking, applying cosmetics or lip balm, and handling contact lenses are prohibited in laboratory work areas.

Food and drink shall not be kept in refrigerators, freezers, shelves, cabinets, or on countertops or bench tops in laboratory areas.

Mouth pipetting/suctioning of blood or other potentially infectious materials is prohibited.

Sharps Management

Contaminated needles and other contaminated sharps shall not be bent, recapped, or removed. Shearing or breaking of contaminated needles is prohibited.

Sharps containers must be closable, puncture resistant, labeled or color-coded red, leak proof on sides and bottom, and maintained upright throughout use. Containers are to be easily accessible to personnel and located as close as is feasible to the immediate area where sharps are used or found. Contaminated disposable sharps shall be discarded, as soon as possible after use, in the disposable sharps containers.

Overfilling of sharps containers creates a hazard when needles protrude from opening. Nearly full containers must be promptly sealed, disposed of appropriately, and replaced by the pharmacist.

Cleaning of Spills, Work Areas, and Equipment

When cleaning up a spill, the following steps will be taken:

- Wear gloves.
- Pick up broken glass, and sharp objects with forceps, tongs, or broom and dust pan
- Wipe up spilled substance using disposable absorbent materials (i.e., paper towels) and discard as contaminated trash.
- Apply 0.5% sodium hypochlorite* (bleach) to the area contaminated by the spill for one minute. Rinse the area thoroughly then dry.
- * A 0.5% sodium hypochlorite solution will be prepared by mixing 1 part 5% stock sodium hypochlorite (commercial bleach) and 9 parts water. A fresh solution should be prepared each day.

Laboratory work surfaces will be decontaminated with 0.5% sodium hypochlorite (bleach) at the completion of each work shift.

Laboratory equipment will be cleaned with 0.5% sodium hypochlorite (bleach) when spillage occurs and when soiled.

Warning Labels

Warning labels shall be affixed to refrigerators and freezers containing blood or other potentially infectious material, and other containers used to store, transport or ship blood or other potentially infectious materials.

These labels shall be fluorescent orange or orange-red or predominantly so, with lettering or symbols in a contrasting color and shall be affixed as close as feasible to the container by string, wire, adhesive, or other method to prevent their loss or unintentional removal.

Personal Protective Equipment

General Guidelines

All required personal protective equipment will be provided, repaired, cleaned, and disposed of by the employer at no cost to the employee. Employees shall wear the appropriate personal protective equipment whenever exposure to skin, eyes, mouth, or other mucous membranes can be reasonably anticipated. Gloves, gowns, and jackets in a variety of sizes as well as face shields, safety glasses, and masks are available. Glove liners or hypoallergenic gloves will be made available to employees who are allergic to the gloves normally provided. All personal protective equipment must be removed before leaving the laboratory.

All tasks or activities that involve handling human specimens require gloves and gown. Any other task or activity that poses a reasonable anticipated risk of splashing requires the use of face protection. Any handling or contact with potentially infectious surfaces (e.g., computer terminals, refrigerator handles, etc.) requires the use of gloves.

The following is a list of typical procedures requiring personal protective equipment. "Gown" means gown or lab jacket; "face protection" means work practice control such as a biosafety shield, a face shield, or safety glasses *and* mask.

Task or Activity	Gloves	Gown	Face Protection
Phlebotomy	Yes	Yes	No
Instrument Operation	Yes	Yes	Recommend if splashback to face is likely

If a protective garment is visibly contaminated by blood or other potentially infectious material, the garment shall be removed as soon as possible and placed in a designated container for laundering or disposal.

Personal protective equipment that will be re-worn shall be kept on a coat hook in the laboratory area when not in use.

Protection for the Hands

Gloves shall be worn in the following situations:

- When it can be reasonably anticipated that hands will contact blood or other potentially infectious material

- When performing finger stick procedures
- When handling or touching contaminated items or surfaces

Disposable Gloves

Replace as soon as feasible when gloves are contaminated, torn, punctured, or when their function as a barrier is compromised.

Do not wash or decontaminate single-use gloves for reuse.

Protection for the Body

Appropriate protective clothing, such as gowns or jackets, are to be worn in occupational exposure situations. The type and characteristic will depend on the task and degree of exposure anticipated.

Hepatitis B Vaccination Policy

All personnel who will have occupational exposure to blood will be offered vaccination against hepatitis B at no cost to the personnel. The vaccination will be administered by an employee health care organization and scheduled by the program director and the involved personnel. All records of dates of vaccination will be maintained by the Program with a photocopy maintained in each employee's personnel file. A signed statement of vaccination refusal will be obtained if the associate declines to be vaccinated. If the employee decides not to receive the vaccine, they will be asked to sign a form stating they were provided the opportunity and received explanation of risk/benefit (Example A).

A pregnancy waiver will be completed as required (Example B).

Procedures for Evaluation and Follow-up of Exposure Incidents

Exposure incidents must be followed up immediately in order to provide prompt treatment if indicated.

In the event of a significant exposure to blood or body fluids (i.e., needle stick, scalpel cuts, blood or body fluid contamination of a cut or scrape, mucous membrane exposure, etc.), testing personnel should immediately wash the affected area with a 5% solution of hypochlorite and then soap and water. The exposure should be reported to the testing personnel's supervisor and an exposure report filled out to document the occurrence within 24 hours (Example C). The pharmacist will have a medical follow-up after the exposure. The medical follow-up will be scheduled with the employee's health care organization by the employee's supervisor. The exposure report and any medical reports will be maintained in the individual associate's records in a

confidential manner. The patient whose blood was involved in the exposure incident will be asked to allow testing of a blood sample for HIV infectivity. The patient will be asked to sign the patient consent or refusal form (Example D). HIV testing will be scheduled by the employee's supervisor.

All laboratory employees are required to inform their supervisor of exposure to potentially hazardous materials as soon as possible after the exposure occurs.

The laboratory shall make available postexposure medical evaluation and follow-up to all employees who have had an exposure incident.

When prophylactic treatment with drugs, vaccines, or immune globulin is deemed necessary and is offered, personnel should be informed of alternative means of prophylaxis, the risk (if this is known) of infection if treatment is not accepted, the degree of protection provided by the therapy, and the potential side effects.

All medical evaluations and procedures are available at no cost to the employee and are made available at a reasonable time and place. All information will be handled in a confidential manner. All procedures will be investigated in a reasonable time. All employees have the right to know the serological status of the source patient. Records will be maintained for 30 years from separation.

An employee exposure report form must be completed within 24 hours of the accident, injury, or event.

Employee Training

Employees will be trained regarding bloodborne pathogens at the time of initial assignment to tasks where exposure may occur and annually, during work hours. Additional training will be provided whenever there are changes in tasks or procedures that affect employees' occupational exposure; this training will be limited to the new exposure situation.

The training approach will be tailored to the educational level, literacy, and language of the employees. The training plan will include an opportunity for employees to have their questions answered by the trainer. The laboratory director or designee is responsible for arranging and/or conducting training. The following training will be provided:

I.   For all new employees *before* they are assigned to an area or activity where occupational exposure exists.

A. The employee will receive task-specific instructions from their supervisor on proper use of protective devices and personal protective equipment. This training will be individualized to ensure understanding.

B. As needed based on the education and training background of the employee, the employee will be provided introductory and background information on how bloodborne pathogens are transmitted and the meaning of "universal precautions." This determination will be the responsibility of the supervisor.

C. Completion of the above will be documented on a personnel training log, reviewed, and signed by the employee and supervisor upon completion. This training log must be completed *before* any occupational exposure exists.

II. The employee's supervisor will provide or arrange for a formalized training program. The program will be attended by all new employees. All existing employees must attend the program annually during the month in which they became employed. The following content will be included in the training:

A. Bloodborne pathogen exposure control plan

B. Universal precautions training

C. Tuberculosis precautions training

D. Bloodborne pathogens standard

E. Epidemiology, modes of transmission, and symptoms of bloodborne diseases

F. Procedures that may expose employees to blood or other potentially infectious materials

G. Control methods that will be used at this facility to prevent/reduce the risk of exposure to blood or other potentially infectious materials

H. Basis for selection of personal protective equipment

I. Hepatitis B vaccination program, including the benefits and safety of vaccination

J. Procedures to use in an emergency involving blood or other potentially infectious materials

K. Procedure to follow if an exposure incident occurs

L. Postexposure evaluation and follow-up procedures

M. Warning labels and/or color coding

N. "Workers Right-to-Know Statement"

Record-Keeping

Training Records

Records documenting all training will be maintained by the employee's supervisor. It is recommended that the records be kept in individual personnel files for easy access (see Appendix I). Training records must be maintained for 3 years. The following information shall be included:

- date of training sessions,
- contents or a summary of the training session,
- name and qualifications of trainer(s), and
- name and job title of all persons attending.

Medical Record-Keeping

A medical record for each employee with exposure will be established and maintained by the laboratory. The record shall be maintained for the duration of employment plus 30 years in accordance with 29 CFR 1910.20.

The record shall include the following:

- name and social security number of the employee;
- a copy of the employee's hepatitis B vaccination status with dates of hepatitis B; vaccinations and any medical records relative to the employee's ability to receive vaccination;
- a copy of examination results, medical testing, and follow-up procedures;
- a copy of the evaluating healthcare professional's written opinion; and
- a copy of the information provided to the healthcare professional who evaluates the employee for suitability to receive hepatitis B vaccination prophylactically and/or after an exposure incident.

The medical record will be kept confidential. The contents will not be disclosed or reported to any person within or outside the workplace without the employee's express written consent, except as required by law or regulation.

Compliance

Failure to comply with this plan will be addressed by the employee's supervisor depending on the severity of the violation.

EXAMPLE A

HEPATITIS B VACCINATION WAIVER FORM

NAME: _____

SOCIAL SECURITY NUMBER: _____

I understand that due to my risk of occupational exposure to blood I may be placing myself at risk of acquiring hepatitis B virus (HBV) infection. I have been given the opportunity by my employer, at no expense to myself, to receive the hepatitis B vaccination series. However, I have decided not to receive the hepatitis B vaccination series. If in the future, I reconsider my decision, I will be given the opportunity to receive the hepatitis B vaccination series at no cost to me.

_____

Signature   Date

_____

Witness' Signature   Date

_____

Witness' Name (Print)

EXAMPLE B

PREGNANCY WAIVER FORM

NAME: _____

SOCIAL SECURITY NUMBER: _____

I understand that due to my risk of occupational exposure to blood I may be placing my child at risk of acquiring hepatitis B virus (HBV) and human immunodeficiency virus (HIV) infections. I have been given the opportunity to stop working with blood. However, I have decided to continue working in situations that may result in exposure to blood. If in the future I reconsider my decision and I am still pregnant, I will be given the opportunity of not working in an area that requires exposure to blood.

_____
Signature   Date

_____
Witness' Signature   Date

_____
Witness' Name (Print)

EXAMPLE C

EXPOSURE REPORT

Postexposure Evaluation and Follow-up

Employee Name: _____

Social Security Number: _____

Date of Exposure: _____

Date Report Filled Out: _____

Describe the circumstances of the exposure:

What was the route of exposure?

List names of witnesses:

Describe HBV and HIV status of source patient, if known:

Describe any medical follow-up:

Copy to: Personnel File

EXAMPLE **D**

Patient Consent or Refusal for
HIV and HBV Infectivity Testing

Patient Name: _____

Date: _____

I understand that health care facilities are required by law to attempt to obtain consent for human immunodeficiency virus (HIV) and hepatitis B virus (HBV) infectivity testing each time a health care worker is
exposed to the blood or bodily fluids OF ANY PATIENT. I understand that a health care worker has been
accidentally exposed to my blood or bodily fluids and that testing for HIV and HBV infectivity is requested. I am not required to give my consent, but if I do, my blood will be tested for these viruses at no
expense to me.

I have been informed that this test can produce a false positive result when an HIV antibody is not
present and that follow-up tests may be required.

I understand that the results of these tests will be kept confidential and will only be released to
medical personnel directly responsible for my care and treatment, to the exposed health care worker for his
or her medical benefit only, and to others only as required by law.

I hereby consent to: I hereby refuse consent to:

❑ HIV testing   ❑ HIV testing

❑ HBV testing   ❑ HBV testing

Signature: _____

(If signed by someone other than patient, please explain relationship.)

Patient Appointment System

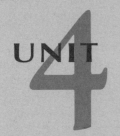

When you are providing patient care services in an ambulatory care setting, a patient appointment system can facilitate care delivery. Depending on your setting, you may be able to utilize a system already in place serving other care providers. If a system is not available, you will need to develop one. This unit will cover the issues related to implementing an appointment system.

Unit Objectives

After you successfully complete this unit, you will be able to:

- explain the benefits of a patient appointment system,
- list factors that affect the time needed to prepare for and conduct patient appointments,
- compare patient appointment systems, and
- describe methods to minimize missed or canceled appointments.

Unit Organization

This unit begins with an explanation of the benefits of a patient appointment system. Factors to consider in determining the length of patient appointments are then described. Next, the length of patient appointments is used to determine hours of operation for the ambulatory patient care service. Systems available to schedule appointments are also compared. Finally, techniques to minimize missed and canceled appointments are presented.

Benefits of a Patient Appointment System

A good appointment system provides many benefits. Such a system:

- improves time management by enabling you to forecast patient load and adjust staffing patterns accordingly;
- allows you to prepare for your interaction and control the time interval of the visit;
- allows you to dedicate uninterrupted time to patients;
- fosters development of a relationship between you and the patient by demonstrating that you dedicate time to patient care;

- facilitates a proactive and preventive approach toward managing the patient's health care needs, including continuous patient monitoring, adherence monitoring, reinforcement, and encouragement; and
- may change patients' expectations and perceptions of pharmacists to more closely match the image of other health care professionals as providers of a service rather than a product.

Allocation of Time for Patient Appointment Activities

You need to allot sufficient time for all patient appointment activities. This avoids overlapping patient appointments and allows time to properly prepare for, conduct, and wrap up the appointment. Make every effort to see patients at their scheduled time and minimize patient waiting time and, thus, dissatisfaction. Factors affecting time allocation and scheduling considerations are discussed below.

Use Your Time Effectively

In the patient care model, pharmacists provide cognitive services directly to the patient. In effect, you are selling your time, not products; keep this in mind as you establish an appointment system. You could easily spend an hour with each patient, but spending a great length of time with an individual patient is not cost-effective. You should set up your services so that the average appointment lasts about 15–20 minutes. This is important to ensure cost-effective service delivery. To be most efficient, try to group patients back-to-back to avoid down time between appointments. Remember, time is money!

Allot approximately 5 minutes to prepare for an initial patient interview, and about 2 minutes for follow-up appointments. Preparation activities may include reviewing the medication profile, reviewing the record and/or medical history form, looking up information about any therapies with which you are unfamiliar, gathering patient education materials and laboratory monitoring supplies and reagents, and preparing a plan of action. Some laboratory equipment, such as the Cholestech cholesterol monitor, must reach room temperature before running tests. The wait can take up to 10 minutes. The time required to run quality control tests on laboratory equipment must also be considered in managing your time. To save time during appointments, run all the necessary controls for tests you will be using at the beginning of the day.

Save time by planning your activities; for example:

- have the patient complete and return a medical history form before the initial visit, so you can review the information ahead of time;
- utilize auxiliary staff to perform tasks such as printing medication profiles for scheduled patients and maintaining stock levels of supplies in the care office;
- use prescription dispensing profiles to determine a rough estimate of patient adherence rates; and
- group patient appointments close enough together so minimal time is wasted between appointments.

Initial Versus Follow-up Appointments

More time is needed for initial appointments because more information is gathered and relayed than at subsequent appointments. During the initial visit, you begin developing patient-pharmacist rapport, you explain your role in the patient's care, and you review the patient's medical history and reasons for being seen. During follow-up visits, you focus on the identification and resolution of pharmacotherapeutic and related health care problems, which generally will not require as much time.

Pharmacist's Skill Level

Initially, appointments will probably last longer than you intend. As you become more proficient, the time needed to conduct an interview and possibly to perform physical assessment, laboratory functions, and documentation will decrease. Be sure to allow a little more time when you first start seeing patients to avoid becoming overwhelmed and running into scheduling problems.

Laboratory Tests

The number of laboratory tests to be performed on a patient will affect not only the time needed for direct interaction with the patient, but also the preparation and possibly follow-up time for an appointment. If performing laboratory monitoring, record the tests you plan to perform at the next visit as part of your plan in the subjective, objective, assessment, plan (SOAP) note and in the appointment scheduling system.

Patient's Health Status

Generally, patients with complicated medication regimens or patients with poorly controlled diseases require more time. Remember to avoid providing the patient with all the information they need to know at one visit. This can be overwhelming to patients and interfere with their ability to retain the information. Overcome the urge to do it all in one visit. While preparing for the appointment and during the interview, determine the most acute problem and focus on that problem with the patient. You can target a different area for the next visit.

Length of Patient Appointment Times

Strive to have the average appointment last 15–20 minutes. You may wish to allow more time initially so you don't become overwhelmed. Adjust the time as you establish your routine and become more comfortable using your skills.

One suggestion is to schedule appointments for 40 minutes when you first start out. Here is a guideline for how you should use this time:

- preparation time: 2–5 minutes (record review and collecting reagents)
- interview time: 20 minutes (question patient, run laboratory tests, record patient responses)
- documentation time: 15 minutes

Administrative Activities

Allot time each workday for administrative activities, such as completing documentation, filing documentation and records, ordering supplies, rescheduling missed appointments, quality assurance monitoring, and making telephone calls.

How to Set Up an Appointment System

Setting up an appointment system requires preparation and can be done in a number of different ways. Decide on a method that will work best in your particular setting, and then make sure everyone affected consistently uses the agreed-on method. Communication between providers in your setting is essential to ensure consistency.

Times of Operation

If you are in a setting in which you have control of hours of operation, choose the times you will offer appointment-based services. Selected times should be based on the resources you have allotted to these services, the availability of staff, and the anticipated patient load. Offering flexibility, such as evening or weekend hours, will help accommodate patient schedules. You need to evaluate the demographics of your potential patient population to determine which hours work best for your patients. Appointments scheduled during regular working hours (9–5) may accommodate retired patients; however, evening and/or weekend hours may be more convenient for individuals who work during the day.

Number of Operating Hours per Week

If you have control of this function, establish hours of operation that correspond to the number of patients you anticipate seeing. Patient loads can be determined based on the time interval you set for patient visits (e.g., every 6–8 weeks), the average time you plan for per patient visit (e.g., 20–30 minutes, including preparation, interview, and documentation time), and subtracting time out of each workday for various administrative activities. Using 7-week intervals between visits and 25 minutes per visit, each patient averages 185.75 minutes per year with the pharmacist. Subtracting 1 hour per day for administrative activities, 4 hours per week can maintain a patient load of 50 patients, whereas 8 hours can maintain a load of 117 patients. A pharmacist devoting 40 hours per week to patient care activities could maintain a practice with 587 patients.

The patient load in the previous example is calculated as follows. If patients are seen on average every 7 weeks, the frequency is equivalent to 7.43 visits per year or 185.75 minutes per patient when the average visit is 25 minutes. The pharmacist devotes 1 hour per day or 3120 minutes per year (52 weeks × 60 minutes) on administrative activities. If the pharmacist allots 4 hours per week to patient care activities, that translates into 3 hours with patients and 1 hour administrative time. Three hours of patient time per week is equivalent to 9360 minutes (180 minutes × 52 weeks) of patient time available per year. Because the average patient utilizes 185.75 minutes of pharmacist time per year, then theoretically each pharmacist could handle a patient population of 50 patients (9360 minutes available per year/185.75 minutes per patient). Correspondingly, if 8 hours per week are devoted to patient care (1 hour administrative activities and 7 hours direct patient care), the theoretical patient load would be 117 (7 hours × 60 minutes × 52 weeks/185.75 minutes per patient).

Methods to Schedule Appointments

The method chosen to schedule appointments is not as important as its consistent use. Several possibilities are discussed below.

Patient Appointment Book

A commercially available appointment book is the easiest and most portable method for scheduling appointments. Designate a particular area to keep the book, so time is not spent searching for it. Consider writing appointments in pencil so they can be changed easily. Use the book to communicate information between different pharmacists providing services and as a reminder of which laboratory test(s) will be performed at the next visit. You can also record any refills the patient will be picking up on that day. This information is useful to provide reminders to patients when you fill out patient appointment cards or when you call patients to confirm appointments. It also lets you prepare needed test reagents and refill prescriptions in advance of the patient's appointment.

Electronic Appointment System

Another option is to schedule appointments using a commercially available computer scheduling program (e.g., Sidekick or Lotus Organizer). This method is not as portable as a book and is more expensive. Many of these systems allow you to add notes regarding a particular appointment, which can be used to document the laboratory tests you wish to perform and any refill information, as you would with a book system. Many systems allow you to print out a daily or weekly calendar of appointments that you can keep posted in the care area.

Use of Support Personnel

Pharmacists are not always available to schedule patient appointments; therefore, support staff should be familiar with the appointment scheduling process. Personnel expected to schedule appointments should receive instruction on scheduling procedures.

Methods to Help Patients Keep Appointments

Many factors can influence patients' ability to attend scheduled appointments. No-shows and cancellations will occur as they do with any appointment-based system. The following techniques can help minimize no-shows and cancellations and help with work flow and staffing patterns as well as save time rescheduling missed appointments.

Schedule Appointments to Accommodate the Patient

You and the patient should decide jointly when and how often to schedule appointments. Involving the patient in the decision-making increases patient satisfaction and results in fewer missed appointments and cancellations.

Schedule appointments when refills are due if you are practicing in a setting that dispenses the patient's prescriptions. The patient will need to come in to pick up refills, and scheduling an appointment to coincide with the refill date will prevent an additional trip. Make every effort to coordinate as many prescription refills as possible with a patient's appointment. Establish a procedure to ensure these prescriptions are filled and ready before the scheduled appointment.

If the patient will be having a laboratory test that requires fasting, schedule the appointment as early in the morning as possible for the patient's comfort and convenience and for reliability of results. The patient's work schedule or transportation availability are other important factors in scheduling appointments that are convenient for patients. You may need to establish evening or weekend hours for patients that cannot be seen during daytime hours.

Appointment Cards

You can use cards similar to those used at physician's or dentist's offices and record the date and time of the next visit. Patients will then have a written reminder of their appointment.

Reminder Cards

Patient reminder postcards can be mailed to patients approximately 1 week in advance of a scheduled appointment. The cards remind patients about their next appointment and any special instructions they may need to follow before the appointment (e.g., fasting before the visit). Using reminder cards avoids

lost time if patients cancel too close to an appointment time and facilitates rescheduling an appointment, if necessary.

Reminder Telephone Calls

Calling the patient 1 or 2 days before his or her scheduled visit to confirm the appointment is useful. The call reminds the patient about the appointment and provides the opportunity to reschedule if there has been a last-minute change in plans. Incorporate these calls into your daily routine by setting aside a time when you will call those patients scheduled for a visit in the next 1 or 2 days. Auxiliary staff can be utilized to fill out and mail reminder cards and make reminder telephone calls.

Communications

You should have a method for patients to schedule or reschedule appointments. An answering machine in the care office can serve this purpose and will also decrease interruptions if you are with other patients. Establish a mechanism to ensure that any communications about patient appointments are duly recorded in your appointment notebook or schedule.

Missed Appointments/Cancellations

Patients should be contacted immediately after missing an appointment. Call to determine the reason for the missed appointment and reschedule at the patient's convenience. Don't reprimand patients for not keeping the appointment, but show concern for their welfare. If the patient is unable to commit to another appointment date, select a future date to contact him or her for rescheduling the appointment. Persistence is necessary with some patients to ensure positive outcomes. Document your attempt to reschedule appointments with the patient.

Summary

The benefits of establishing an appointment system are numerous. A good system allows you to manage time efficiently, anticipate staffing needs, avoid interruptions, improve patient perceptions of the pharmacist's role, and take a proactive approach toward patient management.

Self-Study Questions

Objective

Explain the benefits of a patient appointment system.

1. Which of the following best describes how a patient appointment system benefits time management?

    A. It determines the hours of operation for the ambulatory patient care service.
    B. It allows the pharmacist to take a lunch break.
    C. It allows the pharmacy to adjust staff schedules to accommodate the number of expected patients.
    D. It increases the time that a pharmacist may spend with an individual patient.

2. Describe how a patient appointment system might affect the patient's image of the pharmacist.

Objective

List factors that affect the time needed to prepare for and conduct patient appointments.

3. All of the following need to be considered in determining the length of the appointment *except*:

    A. laboratory test(s) to be conducted.
    B. the skill level of the pharmacist.
    C. the number of operating hours per week.
    D. the complexity of the patient's medication regimen.

4. Which of the following best describes preparation activities?

    A. Laboratory equipment should be prepared at the beginning of the day to minimize wasted time.
    B. Preparing for an appointment usually requires 15–20 minutes.
    C. Documentation consumes most of the time needed for preparation.
    D. Preparation time is the same for initial and follow-up appointments.

5. Describe why the time needed for follow-up appointments is less than the time needed for initial appointments.

Objective

Compare patient appointment systems.

6. Compare the systems used to schedule patient appointments.

Objective

Describe methods to minimize missed or canceled appointments.

7. How can missed or canceled appointments be minimized?

Self-Study Answers

1. C

2. Dedicating uninterrupted time to a patient fosters the patient-pharmacist relationship and demonstrates that the pharmacist is dedicated to patient care. This step may increase the pharmacist's image as a provider of care, not products.

3. C

4. A

5. Initial appointments are often longer because more information is obtained than during follow-up appointments. An explanation of the role of the pharmacist and the establishment of the patient-pharmacist relationship also occur during the initial visit, and this requires additional time.

6. A patient appointment book is inexpensive and easy to use but can be misplaced. An electronic appointment system is more expensive. Both systems can be used to communicate information to other pharmacists or serve to remind the pharmacist of important information.

7. Methods to minimize canceled appointments include scheduling appointments at times that are convenient to the patient (e.g., when the patient has a laboratory test scheduled or needs a medication refill). Use of appointment and reminder cards and reminder telephone calls also minimizes cancellations and missed appointments.

Patient Education Materials

UNIT 5

Patients retain information better when verbal education is supplemented with written materials. Because patients usually cannot remember all the verbal information given to them, written materials help patients remember the key points of an educational session. Written materials can serve as an information resource for patients, caregivers, and family members. Audiovisual materials, audio materials, and demonstration equipment and devices can be used to supplement verbal and written educational materials, depending on the patient's needs and the subject to be addressed. For example, when instructing a patient how to use a metered dose inhaler, a placebo inhaler can be used to supplement verbal instruction.

Unit Objectives

After you successfully complete this unit, you will be able to:

- describe types of patient education materials and state potential sources,
- explain the criteria used to evaluate patient education materials, and
- describe an effective system for organizing and ordering patient education materials.

Unit Organization

To begin, this unit will discuss the scope of patient education materials needed for the ambulatory patient care service. Next, types of patient education materials and potential sources for these materials are discussed. You will then learn how to evaluate these materials based on the guidelines contained in the *Action Plan for the Provision of Useful Patient Information*.[1] The unit concludes with a discussion of a system for ordering and organizing patient education materials.

Types and Availability of Materials

As noted in unit 1, the patient education materials you will require will depend on the type of patients regularly seen in your practice. In addition to having materials that address the needs of your typical patients, you should have a readily available source of materials covering conditions you do not usually see and medications you do not normally use.

Patient education materials are available from many sources, including professional organizations, national disease-specific organizations, pharmaceutical companies, and government agencies. **Table 1** is a list of sources of these materials. This list, while not intended to be exhaustive, should give you an idea of the breadth of sources. Materials may have to be self-developed when a suitable product cannot be found.

A list of materials available can be obtained by calling the sources listed in **Table 1** or pharmaceutical companies and explaining the information you seek. Telephone numbers for the pharmaceutical companies can be found in the *Physician's Desk Reference* and the *Drug Topics Red Book*. If pharmaceutical company representatives call on you or your work site, tell them you want quality materials and describe disease-specific areas of interest. Ask them to keep you informed about new materials. Some patient education materials are free; others have a nominal cost. Some organizations will provide one copy of an educational piece with permission to duplicate as needed.

There are many types of patient education materials: written materials, videotapes, audiotapes, demonstration equipment for specialized dosage forms (e.g., metered dose inhalers, syringes, and practice self-injectors), and demonstration self-monitoring equipment (e.g., peak flow meters and blood glucose monitors). It is a good idea to have a variety of types of materials, because some patients may prefer written materials over videotapes, or vice-versa. In addition, some educational topics are best explained with a videotape rather than in print. For example, a videotape demonstrating how to use a holding chamber for an inhaler may be better reinforcement for an educational session than a written description of how to use the device. A patient's physical limitations (such as limitations in sight or hearing) may dictate the use of specific types of materials (e.g., large-print materials for the visually impaired, Braille or audio materials for the blind, and written materials for the hearing impaired). You also need to consider whether a patient has the equipment to use audiovisual or audio materials at home.

Table 1. Selected Sources of Patient Education Materials

Agency for Health Care Policy and Research
Executive Office Center
2101 East Jefferson Street, Suite 501
Rockville, MD 20852
(800) 358-9295
www.ahcpr.gov

Allergy and Asthma Network
3554 Chain Bridge Road
Suite 200
Fairfax, VA 22030-2709
(800) 878-4403
www.aanma.org

American Cancer Society
1599 Clifton Road NE
Atlanta, GA 30329-4251
(800) 227-2345
www.cancer.org

American College of Obstetricians and Gynecologists
409 12th Street, SW
Washington, DC 20024-2188
(202) 638-5577
www.acog.com

American Diabetes Association
Diabetes Information Service Center
1660 Duke Street
Alexandria, VA 22314-3447
(800) 232-6733
www.diabetes.org

American Dietetic Association
216 West Jackson Boulevard
Chicago, IL 60606-6695
(800) 366-1655
www.eatright.org

American Heart Association
National Center
7272 Greenville Avenue
Dallas, TX 75231-4596
(800) 611-6083
www.americanheart.org

American Lung Association
1740 Broadway
New York, NY 10019-4374
(212) 315-8700
www.lungusa.org

American Menopause Foundation
Madison Square Station
P.O. Box 2013
New York, NY 10010
(212) 714-2398

American Psychiatric Press, Inc.
1400 K Street, NW
Suite 1101
Washington, DC 20005
(800) 368-5777

American Society of Health-System Pharmacists
7272 Wisconsin Avenue
Bethesda, MD 20814
(301) 657-3000
www.ashp.org

Channing L. Bete Co., Inc.
200 State Road
South Deerfield, MA 01373-0200
(800) 628-7733
www.channing-bete.com

Citizens for Public Action on Blood Pressure and Cholesterol, Inc.
7200 Wisconsin Avenue
Suite 1002
Bethesda, MD 20814
(301) 770-1711

Food and Drug Administration
Office of Consumer Affairs
Consumer Inquiries
Information Line
5600 Fishers Lane
Room 16-63 (HFE-88)
Rockville, MD 20857
(800) 535-4555
www.fda.gov

Infodek, Inc.
150 Glenridge Commons
Atlanta, GA 30328
(800) 416-4636

Juvenile Diabetes Foundation
432 Park Avenue South
New York, NY 10016
(800) 533-2873
www.jdfcure.org

Table 1. Selected Sources of Patient Education Materials (cont.)

Medcom, Inc.
P.O. Box 6003
6060 Phyllis Drive
Cypress, CA 90630
(800) 320-1444

National Cancer Institute
Office of Cancer Communications
Building 31, Room 10A24
31 Center Drive MSC 2580
Bethesda, MD 20892-2580
(800) 422-6237
www.nci.nih.gov

**National Council for Patient Information
   and Education**
666 Eleventh Street, NW
Suite 810
Washington, DC 20001
(202) 347-6711

**National Diabetes Information
   Clearinghouse**
Building 31, Room 9A04
9000 Rockville Pike
Bethesda, MD 20892
(301) 654-3327

National Eye Institute
Box 20/20
Bethesda, MD 20892-3665
(800) 869-2020
www.nei.nih.gov

National Heart, Lung, and Blood Institute
NHLBI Information Center
P.O. Box 30105
Bethesda, MD 20884-0105
(301) 251-1222
www.nhlbi.nih.gov/nhlbi/nhlbi.htm

National Institute on Aging
Information Center
P.O. Box 8057
Gaithersburg, MD 20892-8057
(800) 222-2225
www.nih.gov/nia

**National Institute of Diabetes and Digestive
   and Kidney Disease**
31 Center Drive, MSC 2560
Building 31, Room 9A-04
Bethesda, MD 20892-2560
(301) 496-3583

National Institute of Mental Health
Information Resources and Inquiries Branch
Office of Scientific Information
Room 7C-02
5600 Fishers Lane
Rockville, MD 20857
(301) 443-4513

**National Jewish Center for Immunology and
   Respiratory Medicine**
1400 Jackson Street
Denver, CO 80206-2762
(800) 222-5864
www.njc.org

National Mental Health Association
1021 Prince Street
Alexandria, VA 22314-2971
(800) 969-NMHA (6642)
www.nmha.org

National Stroke Association
96 Inverness Drive East, Suite I
Englewood, CO 80112-5112
(303) 649-9299
www.stroke.org

**Nonprescription Drug Manufacturers
   Association**
1150 Connecticut Avenue, NW
Washington, DC 20036
(202) 429-9260
www.ndmainfo.org

The Weight Control Information Network
One Win Way
Bethesda, MD 20892-3665
(301) 951-1120
www.niddk.gov/nutritiondocs.html

Source: adapted from *Ambulatory Care Clinical Skills: Core Module,* unit 16.

Evaluating Patient Education Materials

The *Action Plan for the Provision of Useful Prescription Medicine Information*[1] was developed as the result of a 1996 law passed by Congress requiring the creation of such a plan to improve oral and written communication to patients about their prescription medications. The *Action Plan* recommends guidelines for written patient education materials. Although the guidelines apply to written materials, they can be applied to audiovisual and audio materials as well. Materials should be:

- scientifically accurate,
- unbiased in content and tone,
- sufficiently specific and comprehensive,
- useful,
- timely and up-to-date, and
- presented in an understandable and legible format that is readily comprehensible to consumers.

In the context of these guidelines, "scientifically accurate" means that information about the use of or indications for medications must be consistent with FDA-approved labeling. In the broader context, you must evaluate the content of materials for accuracy of the information presented. The guidelines also say that materials should be "unbiased in tone and content," meaning they should be explanatory; neutral; without comparative adjectives, untruthful claims about the benefit of a product, or hyperbole; and distinguished from any promotional or other information provided to the patient. In addition, the material should present a fair balance between descriptions of risks and benefits. Materials should be "specific and comprehensive" enough to enable patients to use medication correctly, receive maximum benefit, and avoid harm; materials that enable patients to do these things are considered "useful." "Specific and comprehensive" also means the material must provide directions for use and information about avoiding negative consequences. Finally, materials should not contain out-of-date information.

For written materials to be understandable, legible, and readily comprehensible to consumers, the guidelines recommend the use of a large, plain type and a mixture of upper- and lowercase lettering. Type size is very important to readability, and too much curve or detail on a typeface obscures letters and slows reading. Upper- and lowercase letters have more variation in shape and are easier to identify than all uppercase lettering. There should be adequate space between letters, lines, and paragraphs to enhance readability. An eighth-grade or lower reading level is recommended. Important information should be called to the reader's attention with boldface type or by outlining with a box. Important information should not be highlighted or underlined, which can impair readability. Line length should not be too long (i.e., more than approximately 40 letters long). There should be good contrast between ink and paper colors to facilitate reading. Black, dark blue, or brown ink on pale yellow or white paper provides the best contrast. Materials should be printed on uncoated paper. Short paragraphs and bullet points increase readability. Consider avoiding jargon, and use medical terms appropriately. Audiovisual materials should have an appealing presentation and language appropriate for their intended audience. For example, a video on asthma for children would need to use a different presentation style and language level than one for adults.

Before using any written or audiovisual patient education materials in your practice, you should evaluate them, using the above guidelines. **Figure 1** presents a checklist to be used when performing this evaluation. In addition to evaluating materials against the checklist, you should be familiar with the content of the materials you use. Being familiar with the products helps you select the proper one and allows you to address questions that patients may have after using the material.

Ordering and Organizing Materials

Patient education materials must be readily available at the point of care or they will not be used and patients will not benefit. For patient education materials to be used effectively, a system for organizing, filing, stocking, and reordering them must be in place. Time spent organizing and maintaining a system will pay off later.

One person should be designated to be in charge of maintaining set inventory levels of materials, checking in materials when received, and filing in the appropriate place. An example ordering and tracking form is presented in **Figure 2**. This form lists the source of materials, ordering information, title of materials, type of material, inventory

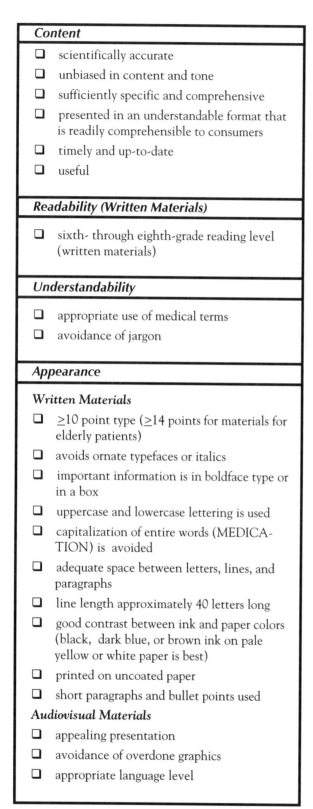

Content

☐ scientifically accurate

☐ unbiased in content and tone

☐ sufficiently specific and comprehensive

☐ presented in an understandable format that is readily comprehensible to consumers

☐ timely and up-to-date

☐ useful

Readability (Written Materials)

☐ sixth- through eighth-grade reading level (written materials)

Understandability

☐ appropriate use of medical terms

☐ avoidance of jargon

Appearance

Written Materials

☐ ≥10 point type (≥14 points for materials for elderly patients)

☐ avoids ornate typefaces or italics

☐ important information is in boldface type or in a box

☐ uppercase and lowercase lettering is used

☐ capitalization of entire words (MEDICA-TION) is avoided

☐ adequate space between letters, lines, and paragraphs

☐ line length approximately 40 letters long

☐ good contrast between ink and paper colors (black, dark blue, or brown ink on pale yellow or white paper is best)

☐ printed on uncoated paper

☐ short paragraphs and bullet points used

Audiovisual Materials

☐ appealing presentation

☐ avoidance of overdone graphics

☐ appropriate language level

Figure 1. Checklist for evaluating written, audio, and audiovisual patient education materials
Source: from reference 2

level, quantity ordered, date ordered, quantity received, and costs. A blank form can be found in **Appendix 1**. A filing cabinet in the care office or close by works well for organizing written materials. Materials can be filed by disease and topic. For example, all materials related to diabetes can be filed together, separated into subtopics such as foot care, diet, medications, etc.

Out-of-Print Materials

Publishers of patient education materials will frequently discontinue printing a particular educational piece. If you find this has happened with one of your favorite patient education materials, ask the publisher if a similar piece is being produced to replace the discontinued item. Always save one copy of educational materials you find particularly useful. If the piece is ever discontinued, you can develop your own educational material from the remaining copy. Be sure to evaluate the content of the original carefully for currency and continued usefulness of the information. Some materials are copyrighted. If you develop your own materials, always give credit to the original source.

Summary

Patient education materials are very important to the patient education process. Depending on your setting, you will need to determine what type of materials you require, set up a system for organizing and ordering the materials, and evaluate all materials before using them.

References

1. Steering Committee for the Colaborative Development of a Long-Range Action Plan for the Provision of Useful Prescription Medicine Information. *Action Plan for the Provision of Useful Prescription Medicine Information.* December 1996. Available at: http://library.nyam.org/keystone. Accessed Dec. 15, 1998.

2. *Ambulatory Care Clinical Skills Program: Core Module.* Bethesda, MD: American Society of Health-System Pharmacists; 1998. Unit 16, Designing patient-specific education. p. 351–71.

Written Patient Education Materials Ordering/Tracking Form

Supplier	Material Title	Inventory Level	Quantity Ordered	Date Ordered	Quantity Received	Date Received	Cost
Information Resources and Inquires Branch, Office of Scientific Information/NIMH, Room 7C-02, 5600 Fishers Lane, Rockville, MD 20857 301-443-4513	**Depression: What Every Woman Should Know** NIH 95-3871	10	20	6/5	20	8/12	
Information Resources and Inquires Branch, Office of Scientific Information/NIMH, Room 7C-02, 5600 Fishers Lane, Rockville, MD 20857 301-443-4513	**Depression: What You Need To Know** NIH 95-3080	15	20	6/5	20	8/12	
Boehringer Mannheim 101 Orchard Ridge Dr. Gaithersburg, MD 20878 301-216-3545	Diabetes Management Diary	20	20	7/8	20	9/15	

Figure 2. Example Ordering and Tracking Form
Source: adapted from reference 2

Self-Study Questions

Objective

Describe types of patient education materials and state potential sources.

1. Describe how a patient's physical limitations might affect the type of educational material chosen.

2. All of the following are potential sources of patient education materials *except:*

    A. drug manufacturers.
    B. government agencies.
    C. pharmacy schools.
    D. national associations.

Objective

Explain the criteria used to evaluate patient education materials.

3. Which of the following defines criteria to evaluate the format of patient education materials?

    A. Omnibus Reconciliation Act of 1990
    B. *Action Plan for the Provision of Useful Patient Information*
    C. the state pharmacy practice act
    D. Freedom of Information Act

4. List elements of patient education materials that need to be evaluated.

Objective

Describe an effective system for organizing and ordering patient education materials.

5. All of the following describe a system for ordering and organizing patient education materials *except:*

    A. The system ensures that materials will be available when needed.
    B. One person should be designated to maintain and order patient education materials.
    C. Set inventory levels are used to determine the order quantity.
    D. A properly run system can decrease the cost of the patient education program.

Self-Study Answers

1. A patient's physical limitations may require the use of specialized educational materials. For example, patient's with vision limitations may require written information with large-print and patients with hearing loss may not be able to use audio materials.

2. C

3. B

4. A review of patient educational materials should include an evaluation of content, readability, and appearance of the material.

5. D

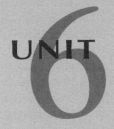

UNIT
Documentation

Documentation is an essential part of providing patient care services. As pharmacists take on expanded roles in providing health services, documentation will become even more important.

A good documentation system:
- facilitates your interactions with patients,
- facilitates provision of pharmaceutical care and assurance of optimal outcomes,
- provides necessary documentation for reimbursement of cognitive services, and
- provides necessary legal documentation.

Maintaining good records helps you provide quality patient care services. Adequate documentation avoids the need to repeat questions and information from previous patient interactions, helps save time, and establishes a good pharmacist-patient relationship. Having information recorded and stored in an easily accessible manner assists you in providing pharmaceutical care and helps ensure desired outcomes by allowing easy tracking of patients. As you provide direct patient care services and expect to be paid for them, payers of your services will expect documentation of the services provided and the outcomes. If a question ever arises about the details of your patient interaction or professional judgment, a good documentation system will facilitate the evaluation process. Just because you have kept records for your purposes does not mean these records could not or will not be used at some time in a legal case against you or another health care provider.

Unit Objectives

After you successfully complete this unit, you will be able to:
- describe elements of a documentation system;
- explain the documentation process, including the use of the SOAP (subjective, objective, assessment, plan) note;
- describe the importance of communicating with other health care providers and list methods of communication; and
- describe methods to organize and maintain patient records.

Unit Organization

Unit 6 begins with a discussion of areas of patient care that require documentation, and example forms

for gathering and recording this information are provided. Next, the SOAP note is used to demonstrate information required in a pharmacist's care notes. Methods to communicate important findings to the patient's other health care providers are then described. Finally, systems for maintaining and organizing patient records are explored.

Areas of Documentation

The major areas of documentation are:
- consent forms,
- patient information,
- therapy assessment and monitoring,
- pharmacist's care plans,
- patient interactions, and
- communications with other health care providers.

This unit will focus primarily on the documentation issues pertaining to patient information, therapy assessment and monitoring, care plans, interactions, and communication with other health care practitioners. Refer to unit 10, Legal Issues, for information on the use of consent forms.

Gathering Patient Information

To define and solve patient-specific pharmacotherapeutic and related health care problems, you need to collect and document a significant amount of information about a patient. To do this in an efficient manner that organizes the information in a usable format, you should use some type of data collection form. A form will ensure that you do not miss collecting any pertinent information and will allow you to easily retrieve the information when needed.

For example, you are seeing Sarah Mistler, a 58-year-old woman, in your diabetes clinic. She is having difficulty controlling her diabetes. An example of a database form, the Pharmacist's Patient Database Form, used for collecting information in an ambulatory care setting for Mrs. Mistler is given in **Figure 1**. This form collects demographic, administrative, medical, drug therapy, behavioral/lifestyle, and social/economic information about a patient. A blank copy of this form can be found in **Appendix 1**.

Assessing Therapy

Once you have collected information about patients, you will assess their therapy and document

PHARMACIST'S PATIENT DATABASE FORM

Original Date: _1/13/98_
Date updated:_____
Date updated:_____
Date updated:_____

Demographic and Administrative Information

Name: **Sarah Mistler**

Social Security #: **123-45-6789**

Address: **Rt. 1, Box 485, Stony Brook, VA   23478**

Health Care Provider's Name **Jim Belvin**

Health Care Provider's Phone **200-0001**

Work Phone: Home Phone:

Date of Birth: **01/04/40**

Race: **White**

Gender: **Female**

Religion: **Methodist**

Occupation: **Factory worker**

Health Insurer: **BC/BS of VA**

Subscriber #: **3561789592**

Primary Card Holder: **same**

Drug Benefit: ☒ yes   ☐ no   copay: $ **5/10**

Current Symptoms

1/13 - denies s/s of hypo, hyperglylcemia or complications

Past Medical History	Acute and Current Medical Problems
Hysterectomy at age 40	1. HTN
w/ oophorectomy	2. Type II diabetes
h/o frequent vaginal fungal infections	3. Hypercholesterolemia
h/o diabetic foot ulcer 6/97	4.
h/o hospitalization for pneumonia 12/96	5.
	6.
	7.

Family/Social/Economic History	Personal Limitations
Lives w/retired husband, 4 children	none
(1 still lives w/her) mother died -	
breast cancer @ 72, father died - MI @ 50	
Cost of medications per month $_____	

Allergies/Intolerances

☐ No known drug allergies

Medication	Reaction
codeine	N, V, rash
meperidine	hallucinations

Social Drug Use

Alcohol	occasional beer
Caffeine	3 cups coffee/day
Tobacco	1 1/2 packs/day

Pregnancy/Breastfeeding Status

☐ Pregnant (due _____)   ☐ Breastfeeding

Diet	Routine Exercise/Recreation	Daily Activities/Timing
☒ Low salt prescribed	no routine exercise	works 7a - 3:30p shift
☒ Low fat supposed to be on	Cleans house and works	gets up at 4:30a
☒ Diabetic but not following	in garden on wkends	goes to bed at 9:30p
Timing of meals: B: 5:30a, L: 12noon, D: 5p		

Figure 1. Pharmacist's Patient Database Form for Mrs. Mistler

Patient Name: **Sarah Mistler**

Physical Assessment/Laboratory Data—Initial/Follow-up

Date	1/13/98				
Height	5'4"				
Weight	174 lbs				
Temp					
BP	Ⓡ 158/96, 160/96 Ⓛ				
Pulse	72 regular				
Respirations					
Peak Flow					
FBG					
R. Glucose	210				
HgbA$_{1c}$	10%				
T. Chol.	250				
LDL					
HDL					
TG					
INR					
BUN					
Cr					
ALT					
AST					
Alk Phos					

Drug Serum Concentrations

Date					

Notes: 1/13 - Has good understanding of medications. Does not self-monitor glucose→ MD wants her to start

Figure 1. Pharmacist's Patient Database Form for Mrs. Mistler (continued)

Patient Name: Sarah Mistler

Current Prescription Medication Regimen

Name/Dose/Strength/Route	Schedule/Frequency of Use	Indication	Start Date (and stop date if applicable)	Prescriber	Adherence Issues/Efficacy
Metformin 500mg	TID w/meals	diabetes	a year ago	Belvin	Rarely misses dose
HCTZ 50mg	9am	HTN	1989	"	"
Cholestyramine 1 pkt	TID (spaced from other meds)	Cholesterol	1989	"	Difficulty
EC Aspirin 325 mg	9am	MI prevention	1990	"	

Current Nonprescription Medication Regimen (OTC, herbal, homeopathic, nutritional, etc.)

Name/Dose/Strength/Route	Schedule/Frequency of Use	Indication	Start Date (and stop date if applicable)	Prescriber	Adherence Issues/Efficacy
Acetaminophen 500mg	1-2 tabs x 1	headache (~1/wk)			usually works
Ibuprofen 200mg	2 tabs	headache (if above doesn't work)			works
Valerian (?brand/strength) 1 cap		sleep (2-3/week)	1/98		helps

Figure 1. Pharmacist's Patient Database Form for Mrs. Mistler (continued)

Patient Name: __Sarah Mistler__

Risk Assessment/Preventive Measures/Quality of Life

Cardiovascular Risk Assessment		
male > 45 years old	1	—
female > 55 years old or female < 55 with history of ovarectomy not taking estrogen replacement	1	1
Definite MI or sudden death before age 55 year in father or male first-degree relative or before 65 year in mother or female first-degree relative	1	—
current cigarette smoking	1	1
hypertension	1	1
diabetes mellitus	1	1
HDL cholesterol < 35 mg/dl	1	Need HDL to complete
HDL cholesterol > 60 mg/dl	-1	
	TOTAL:	

Is patient at risk for complications of current conditions?   ☒ Yes   ☐ No
Specify:
     Need more information

Preventive Measures for Adults
H = has been done   R = patient refuses   X = not applicable   Date

Women		1997			
Pap Smear/pelvic	Annually 19+	H			
Mammogram	Every 1-2Y 40-49; annually 50+	H			
Men					
Rectal/prostate	Annually 50+				
All Patients					
Total/HDL-C	Every 5Y 19+	H			
Home Fecal Occult Blood Test	Annually	H			
Immunizations					
Td	Every 10Y	H			
Influenza	Every fall*	H			
Pneumovax	Once*	H			

* if indicated

Quality of life issues

Figure 1. Pharmacist's Patient Database Form for Mrs. Mistler (continued)

Ambulatory Therapy Assessment Worksheet (ATAW)

Patient _Sarah Mistler_

Pharmacist _Susanne Webster_

Date _1-13-98_

Correlation Between Drug Therapy and Medical Problems

ASSESSMENT	PRESENCE OF PROBLEM*	COMMENTS/NOTES
Any drugs without a medical indication? Any unidentified medications? Any untreated medical conditions? Do they require drug therapy?	1. A problem exists. 2. More information is needed for determination. ③ No problem exists or an intervention is not needed.	

Appropriate Therapy

ASSESSMENT	PRESENCE OF PROBLEM*	COMMENTS/NOTES
Comparative efficacy of chosen medication(s)? Relative safety of chosen medication(s)? Is medication on formulary? Is nondrug therapy appropriately used (e.g., diet and exercise)? Is therapy achieving desired goals or outcomes? Is therapy tailored to this patient (e.g., age, comorbid conditions, and living/working environment)?	① A problem exists. 2. More information is needed for determination. 3. No problem exists or an intervention is not needed.	Reconsider use of HCTZ due to possible adverse effects on BG & lipids. Consider exercise therapy. HTN, DM, & cholesterol under poor control.

Drug Regimen

ASSESSMENT	PRESENCE OF PROBLEM*	COMMENTS/NOTES
Are dose and dosing regimen appropriate and/or within usual therapeutic range and/or modified for patient factors? Appropriateness of PRN medications (prescribed or taken that way) Is route/dosage form/mode of administration appropriate, length or course of therapy considering efficacy, safety, convenience, patient limitations, length or course of therapy, and cost?	① A problem exists. 2. More information is needed for determination. 3. No problem exists or an intervention is not needed.	If patient continues on HCTZ, consider ↓ dose to 25 mg.

*Problem denotes any pharmacotherapeutic or related health care problem.

Figure 2. Ambulatory Therapy Assessment Worksheet (ATAW) for Mrs. Mistler

Therapeutic Duplication

ASSESSMENT	PRESENCE OF PROBLEM*	COMMENTS/NOTES
Any therapeutic duplications?	1. A problem exists. 2. More information is needed for determination. ③ No problem exists or an intervention is not needed.	

Drug Allergy or Intolerance

ASSESSMENT	PRESENCE OF PROBLEM*	COMMENTS/NOTES
Allergy or intolerance to any medications (or chemically related medications) currently being taken? Is patient using a method to alert health care providers of the allergy/intolerance or serious health problem?	1. A problem exists. 2. More information is needed for determination. ③ No problem exists or an intervention is not needed.	Allergy to codeine noted.

Adverse Drug Events

ASSESSMENT	PRESENCE OF PROBLEM*	COMMENTS/NOTES
Are symptoms or medical problems drug induced? What is the likelihood the problem is drug related?	1. A problem exists. 2. More information is needed for determination. ③ No problem exists or an intervention is not needed.	

Interactions: Drug-Drug, Drug-Disease, Drug-Nutrient, Drug–Laboratory Test

ASSESSMENT	PRESENCE OF PROBLEM*	COMMENTS/NOTES
Any drug-drug interactions? Clinical significance? Any relative or absolute contraindications given patient characteristics and current/past disease states? Any drug-nutrient interactions? Clinical significance? Any drug-laboratory test interactions? Clinical significance?	① A problem exists. 2. More information is needed for determination. 3. No problem exists or an intervention is not needed.	HCTZ can negatively impact control of DM & hyperlipidemia. Be aware of possible ↑ in BP 2° to NSAIDs. ↑

*Problem denotes any pharmacotherapeutic or related health care problem.

Figure 2. Ambulatory Therapy Assessment Worksheet (ATAW) for Mrs. Mistler (continued)

Social or Recreational Drug Use

ASSESSMENT	PRESENCE OF PROBLEM*	COMMENTS/NOTES
Is current use of social drugs problematic? Are symptoms related to sudden withdrawal or discontinuation of social drugs?	(1) A problem exists. 2. More information is needed for determination. 3. No problem exists or an intervention is not needed.	*Encourage discontinuation of smoking.*

Financial Impact

ASSESSMENT	PRESENCE OF PROBLEM*	COMMENTS/NOTES
Is therapy cost-effective? Does cost of therapy represent a financial hardship for the patient?	1. A problem exists. 2. More information is needed for determination. (3) No problem exists or an intervention is not needed.	

Patient Knowledge of Therapy

ASSESSMENT	PRESENCE OF PROBLEM*	COMMENTS/NOTES
Does patient understand the role of his/her medication(s), how to take it, and potential side effects? Would patient benefit from education tools (e.g., written patient education sheets, wallet cards, or reminder package?) Does the patient understand the role of nondrug therapy?	1. A problem exists. 2. More information is needed for determination. (3) No problem exists or an intervention is not needed.	

Adherence

ASSESSMENT	PRESENCE OF PROBLEM*	COMMENTS/NOTES
Is there a problem with nonadherence to drug or nondrug therapy (e.g., diet and exercise)? Are there barriers to adherence or factors hindering the achievement of therapeutic efficacy?	(1) A problem exists. 2. More information is needed for determination. 3. No problem exists or an intervention is not needed.	*Unable to comply with midday dose of cholestyramine at work.* *Poor adherence with diabetic, low-fat, and low-salt diets.*

*Problem denotes any pharmacotherapeutic or related health care problem.

Figure 2. Ambulatory Therapy Assessment Worksheet (ATAW) for Mrs. Mistler (continued)

Self-Monitoring

ASSESSMENT	PRESENCE OF PROBLEM*	COMMENTS/NOTES
Does patient perform appropriate self-monitoring? (e.g., peak flow and blood glucose) Is correct technique employed? Is self-monitoring performed consistently, at appropriate times, and with appropriate frequency?	(1) A problem exists. 2. More information is needed for determination. 3. No problem exists or an intervention is not needed.	*Currently not performing home glucose monitoring.*

Risks and Quality of Life Impacts

ASSESSMENT	PRESENCE OF PROBLEM*	COMMENTS/NOTES
Is patient at risk for complications with an existing disease state (i.e., risk factor assessment)? Is patient on track for preventive measures (e.g., immunizations, mammograms, prostate exams, eye exams)? Is therapy adversely impacting patient's quality of life? How so?	1. A problem exists. (2) More information is needed for determination. 3. No problem exists or an intervention is not needed.	*Assess HDL value.* *Need to determine if patient is receiving recommended monitoring for diabetes.* *Need to assess impact of therapy on QOL.*

*Problem denotes any pharmacotherapeutic or related health care problem.

Figure 2. Ambulatory Therapy Assessment Worksheet (ATAW) for Mrs. Mistler (continued)

your assessment. An example tool, the Ambulatory Therapy Assessment Worksheet (ATAW), for assessing patient's therapy using Mrs. Mistler's information is given in **Figure 2** (page 89). The ATAW provides a systematic approach to evaluating a patient's pharmacotherapeutic regimen and non-drug therapy with the goal of establishing a Therapy Problem List.[1] The use of a systematic process helps ensure the generated problem list is complete and takes into account everything you should consider when setting pharmacotherapeutic and related health care goals for each identified problem.[1] Using guiding questions, the ATAW prompts you to consider all possible problem areas.[1] A blank version of this tool can be found in **Appendix 1**.

Documenting Your Plan for Patients

A good way to document not only your final assessment of a patient's therapy but also your plan for intervention is an Ambulatory Pharmacist's Care Plan (APCP). An example plan for Mrs. Mistler is given in **Figure 3**; a blank plan is included in **Appendix 1**.

The pharmacist's care plan serves several important purposes for the ambulatory care pharmacist. The care plan documents an individualized strategy to provide pharmaceutical care for a specific patient. The plan provides a systematic evaluation of the patient so all important problems are considered and followed up, provides an efficient roadmap for providing care, and serves as a communication tool between pharmacists providing care for the same patient. Based on patient-, disease-, and drug-specific data, your plan states pharmacotherapeutic and related health care goals, a strategy to achieve them, and a means to measure their achievement. This plan also serves as a reference when you recommend therapy to the patient, the patient's family, and other health care providers.[2]

Monitoring Your Plan

To provide optimal therapy (i.e., pharmaceutical care) once you have instituted your care plan for a patient, you must continually monitor the patient's progress toward the goals established in the plan. This monitoring can be facilitated by using a consistent process. An example monitoring form, the Ambulatory Monitoring Worksheet (AMW), is completed for Mrs. Mistler in **Figure 4**. This worksheet is the tool that allows you to track your patient's progress and

the outcomes of your therapy recommendations. A blank copy of this form can be found in **Appendix 1**.

Additional information about utilization of each of the previously mentioned forms can be found in the *Ambulatory Care Clinical Skills Program: Core Module*. These forms are tools to support patient care delivery by organizing information in a retrievable format and by facilitating recognition of trends and changes in patient status.

Documenting Interactions with Patients

Pharmacist notes document a patient's problems, your assessment of the problems, the plan you have formulated to address the problems, and the outcomes. Pharmacist notes serve as a permanent record of your interactions. They track your thoughts and actions in the patient care process. They can be used to justify your services, receive payment for services, and may be helpful in legal situations. You will rely on your notes to prepare for each patient appointment, to target interventions, and to assess how well your plan is working. Good notes facilitate the care process and the continuity of care, and they save time. This documentation is essential if your patients see other health care providers who have access to your notes. Your colleagues will be able to quickly determine where you are in the care process with a particular patient and pick up where you left off.

Items that *must* routinely be documented in pharmacist's notes include:

- patient interactions (in person and via telephone);
- objective measurements (e.g., blood pressure readings and laboratory values);
- recommendations and instructions;
- educational instruction and materials provided to patients;
- follow-up with patients who failed to show for appointments; and
- termination of relationship with a patient.

Pharmacist notes should be completed in a timely fashion. The longer you wait before documenting your thoughts, the more likely you are to omit important information. As you see additional patients or speak with other health care providers, the information may tend to blend together. Having notes accumulate can be overwhelming. The best time to complete the note is during or right after the interaction. If this is not possible, complete it as soon after the interaction as possible.

Ambulatory Pharmacist's Care Plan

Patient ___Sarah Mistler___   Pharmacist ___Susanne Webster___   Date ___1/13/98___

DATE IDENTIFIED	PROBLEM (TPL)	PHARMACOTHERAPEUTIC AND RELATED HEALTH CARE GOAL	RECOMMENDATIONS FOR THERAPY	MONITORING PARAMETER(S)	DESIRED ENDPOINT(S)	MONITORING FREQUENCY
1-13-98	Poor control of diabetes	Improve control of diabetes	d/c HCTZ HGM to gain pattern of glucose control Determine MD endpoints	self-monitoring record FBG HgbAlC	Daily monitoring FBG:80-120 mg/dl HgbAlC: <7%	Self-monitoring q visit FBG q 3-4 visits HgbAlC q 6 mo
1-13-98	Poor control of HTN	Improve control of HTN	Δ HCTZ to enalapril 10 mg qd	BP	<135/85 unless otherwise specified	Each visit (q2-4 wks following change in therapy)
1-13-98	Poor control of cholesterol	Improve cholesterol control	d/c cholestyramine start lovastatin 10 mg q evening d/c HCTZ	Lipid profile TC	LDL < 130 mg/dl TC < 200 mg/dl	Lipid profile 2x/year TC—each visit
1-13-98	Potential for HCTZ to adversely affect lipids & DM	Avoid adverse effects of medications	d/c HCTZ	Pt. profile and interview	Pt. no longer on HCTZ	At each visit until resolved
1-13-98	Smoking	Stop smoking	Address at later date due to patient resistance	Pt. interview	Pt. agrees to smoking cessation	4x/yr
1-13-98	No exercise	Start exercise program	MD recommendation for exercise	Pt. interview	Pt. starts exercise plan	Each visit
1-13-98	No home glucose monitoring	Start home glucose monitoring	Monitor fasting glucose daily	Pt. interview Pt. demonstration	Daily monitoring Appropriate technique	→Each visit →2x/year
1-13-98	Adherence problem w/ cholestyramine	Improve adherence with cholestyramine	d/c cholestyramine	Pt. profile Pt. interview	Pt. no longer on cholestyramine	Each visit until resolved

continued ⟶

Figure 3. Ambulatory Pharmacist's Care Plan for Mrs. Mistler

Ambulatory Pharmacist's Care Plan

Patient Sarah Mistler   Pharmacist Susanne Webster   Date 1/13/98

DATE IDENTIFIED	PROBLEM (TPL)	PHARMACOTHERAPEUTIC AND RELATED HEALTH CARE GOAL	RECOMMENDATIONS FOR THERAPY	MONITORING PARAMETER(S)	DESIRED ENDPOINT(S)	MONITORING FREQUENCY
1-13-98	Poor adherence w/ diabetic, low-salt, low-fat diet	Improve adherence with diet	Pt. education and refer to dietitian if necessary	Pt. interview → Weight →	Diet adherence 10% loss	Each visit

Figure 3. Ambulatory Pharmacist's Care Plan for Mrs. Mistler (continued)

PHARMACIST'S CARE PLAN AMBULATORY MONITORING WORKSHEET (AMW)

Patient __Sarah Mistler__   Pharmacist __Susanne Webster__
Date __1-13-98__

Pharmaco-therapeutic Goal	Monitoring Parameter	Desired Endpoint	Monitoring Frequency	1/13	2/10	4/7	5/19	8/21						
1	Glucose self-monitoring record	FB: 80-120 mg/dl	each visit		✓			✓						
1	HgbAIC	<7%	q6mo	10%				7.5%						
1	FBG	80-120 mg/dl	q3-4 visits		225	190	155	146						
2	BP	<135/85	Each visit	160/96	158/92	145/90	140/88	138/86						
3	Lipid profile	LDL <130 mg/dl	twice/yr		T=248 L=165 H=40			T=220 L=144 H=40						
3	Total cholesterol	TC < 200 mg/dl	Each visit	250 ↑	240 ↑	230 ↑								
4	Patient interview and profile	Pt. no longer on HCTZ	Each visit until resolved			Resolved								
5	Patient interview	Pt. agrees to smoking cessation	4x/year		✓									
6	Patient interview	Pt. starts exercise program	Each visit		✓	✓	✓							
7	Patient interview	Daily BG monitoring	Each visit		✓	✓	✓							
7	Patient demo of monitor technique	Appropriate technique	twice/yr		✓									
8	Patient profile and interview	Pt. no longer on cholestyramine	Each visit until resolved		✓			Resolved						
9	Patient interview	Diet adherence	Each visit		✓	✓	✓	✓						

continued →

Figure 4. Monitoring Worksheet for Mrs. Mistler

PHARMACIST'S CARE PLAN AMBULATORY MONITORING WORKSHEET (AMW)

Patient Sarah Mistler

Pharmacist Susanne Webster

Date 1-13-98

Pharmaco-therapeutic Goal	Monitoring Parameter	Desired Endpoint	Monitoring Frequency	Date														
				1/13	2/10	4/7	5/19	8/21									
9	Weight	10% weight loss	Each visit	174	173	169	162	157									

Figure 4. Monitoring Worksheet for Mrs. Mistler (continued)

Initially, writing notes can be time consuming. Don't be overwhelmed. With practice you will develop a consistent style, and the time required for note writing will decrease.

You should use a standardized format, such as the SOAP (subjective, objective, assessment, plan) format, to write your notes. A standardized format ensures consistency in the type of information recorded and facilitates the retrieval and review of information. If all providers use a similar format, each one will know where to find information regardless of who wrote the note.

The SOAP format is recommended because it is recognized by nearly all health professionals. When speaking with physicians, it is helpful to provide the information in this format because they expect to hear the information in that order.

Writing Pharmacist Notes Using the SOAP Format

The following guidelines are provided to help you write notes in the SOAP format. An example SOAP note for a visit with Mrs. Mistler is provided in **Figure 5**.

General Information

Document the date and time of each patient interaction.

Subjective Information

Subjective information is what patients relate to you about their condition that is not readily observable or quantifiable. For example, symptoms such as nausea and dizziness are subjective because they are experienced by the patient but cannot be measured objectively. There are several items documented in this section of the note:

- patient's comments on general well-being;
- patient's primary complaint/concern and any other complaints;
- comments on adherence to medication and nondrug therapies;
- changes in medication regimen (nonprescription and prescription);
- adverse effects of medications the patient is experiencing;
- home monitoring, including frequency of monitoring and results; and
- any changes made at the last physician visit.

Objective Information

Objective information is quantifiable, observable, or obtained in an unbiased manner. Objective information includes physical assessment information and results of any laboratory or diagnostic testing (e.g.,

blood pressure monitoring, cholesterol results, weight, etc.).

Assessment

In this section of the note, document your assessment or impression of the patient's condition based on the subjective and objective information you have gathered. Identify the patient's problems and what may have caused them. Your assessment serves as the basis for formulating your plan and recommendations. The information you should document in this section includes:

- a summary of patient complaints;
- a comparison of patient complaints and objective measurements with previous visits;
- possible causes of complaints;
- objective and subjective measurements that validate your assessment;
- assessment of the patient's adherence to his or her treatment plan;
- regimen review, with identification of pharmacotherapeutic and related health care problems; and
- an assessment of the patient's knowledge and understanding of his or her disease, therapy, and monitoring.

Plan

The plan is targeted at correcting the problems identified during your assessment. Determine what actions you need to take for each problem identified and document those actions you implement at the appointment and those that require follow-up at future appointments.

Note-Writing Tips

Writing notes may seem overwhelming when you first start this process. Initially you may want to document everything, for fear you will forget something. Your initial notes may be long but will become more concise as you become more familiar with your patients and with the process. Here are some note-writing tips:

- Record pertinent positive and negative findings.
- Be correct and complete.
- Use concise wording.
- Do *not* expand on irrelevant data.
- Focus on any changes from the patient's baseline status.
- Do not use inflammatory or accusatory language and/or tone.

5/19/98

Mrs. Sarah Mistler
Date of Birth: Jan. 4, 1940

Subjective:

During the past month, the patient has generally been doing better, and the control of her diabetes has improved. She saw the dietitian and has enthusiastically implemented multiple dietary changes. Is up to walking 4 days per week for 20 minutes at a time. Denies missing any doses of medications. Denies adverse effects from her medications or symptoms of any of her conditions.

Home fasting glucose is averaging 160.

Objective:

Fasting Blood Sugar 155
Fasting Lipid Profile
    Total Cholesterol 230 mg/dl
    LDL   150
    HDL   55
    Triglycerides   75
Pulse   72 bpm, reg
Blood Pressure-1
    140/88 (24 hours post med., left arm)
Blood Pressure-2
    140/88 (24 hours post med., left arm)
Weight   162 lb

Assessment & Plan:

Patient is continuing to progress toward her goals. Praised patient for all her good work. She agreed to increase her walking to 6 days per week. Will continue with daily FBG monitoring at home. Will send an update letter to Dr. Belvin to let him know her progress. Next physician appointment is 7/21/98. Next pharmacist appointment was scheduled for 8/1/98.

Susanne Webster, R.Ph.

Figure 5. Example SOAP note for Mrs. Mistler

Communications with Physicians or Other Health Care Providers

In provision of direct patient services, pharmacists obtain information that can be very useful to other health care professionals involved in a patient's care. Communication of this information serves to:

- share valuable information regarding a patient's medication usage and outcomes with the health care provider responsible for the patient's care (as well as other providers);
- help the pharmacist develop a relationship with the patient's primary physician and become an integral part of the health care team;
- promote the concept that by analyzing the patient's pharmacotherapeutic and related health care problems and recommending therapeutic and monitoring plans, the probability of attaining the desired outcomes will be maximized; and
- assist the pharmacist in solving the patient's pharmacotherapeutic and related health care problems.

If you are in a setting where the physician or other health care provider does not have access to your notes, letters provide a nonthreatening means to share information and discuss chronic problems. Establishing a standardized format for these letters saves time and ensures consistency in the communications.

Letters may be written to inform the health care provider of your activities and the patient's medication use, solve chronic pharmacotherapeutic and related health care problems, follow up when the health care provider has referred the patient to you for a specific reason, follow up when the health care provider has initiated your recommendations, and refer the patient to another health care provider for a specific service. Routine recommendations (e.g., to decrease or increase dose, to add or discontinue medications, to use alternative medication, to request laboratory monitoring, etc.) can be made through a letter. State clearly the reasons for your recommendation and present information that justifies your conclusions. This specific information allows the physician to review your clinical information and incorporate it into his or her plans when seeing the patient.

When a health care provider has initiated your recommendations, a letter serves as a progress report to share information about how the patient is responding to the change in therapy. A letter can be used to refer the patient to another provider, in which case you would provide the background information about the patient. For example, you may wish to refer a patient to a dietitian. You would provide background about the patient's current diet and weight, target goals, strategies you have already utilized with the patient, and the reason for the referral.

In writing letters, be clear, concise, and credible. The information presented may be used to make clinical decisions, so it must be accurate. If you are making recommendations, provide information that will justify or explain your conclusions.

You will not need to write letters after each patient appointment. Do not overwhelm other providers with needless communication. You will make a much greater impact with a few well-written and timely letters.

The elements of a letter include:
- your address and phone number;
- the date;
- an introductory paragraph;
- pertinent background information, including current prescription and nonprescription medications as well as assessment of the degree of adherence to medication regimens and nondrug therapy;
- recent objective measurements;
- a list of problems that you are working on with the patient, strategies you are using to solve these problems, and your assessment of the patient's progress toward his or her goals;
- a list of problems that require action, with the rationale for your recommendations; and
- a concluding paragraph.

An example of a letter sent to Mrs. Mistler's physician is given in **Figure 6**.

Telephone conversations concerning patients should be documented. The documentation of patient-related telephone conversations should contain the following information:
- date and time of telephone conversation,
- name of health care provider with whom you had the conversation,
- items discussed, and
- action taken.

An example of a telephone conversation about Mrs. Mistler is provided in **Figure 7**.

Maintaining Patient Records

You need to develop a record system for organizing all the documents previously discussed, unless your setting already has such a system. This section will review the procedures for setting up and maintaining a record system.

There are two major options for patient record systems: hard copy and electronic systems. Hard copy records are inexpensive and can be tailored to the individual setting. A disadvantage is the time necessary to correctly file information, the need for storage space, and the difficulty retrieving information if standard data collection forms are not used. Advantages of an electronic system include standardized data collection, generation of reports, easy retrieval of information, compact storage, and increased efficiency. The generation of reports and easy retrieval of information facilitates data collection for medication use evaluations, quality assurance monitoring, and research studies. For example, with some systems you can search for all your patients on digoxin and their most recent potassium and digoxin serum concentrations.

If you use an electronic medical record system, you need to have a back-up system, in the event something happens to the electronic files. This can be either electronic back-ups of the data or hard copy records of your electronic notes.

Record Organization

Set up standard procedures for organizing material within each hard copy record and for filing the records. Use of a standardized format facilitates timely retrieval of information when needed.

The following is one suggested way to arrange documents within the record. The most important point is that each person using the records files the documents in the same order. On the left side of the record, file documents such as:
- the patient database,
- therapy assessment forms,
- care plans,
- monitoring worksheets, and
- patient release statements.

These documents will then be readily accessible for reviewing and updating as needed.

On the right side of the record, file documents pertaining to each patient interaction and communication regarding the patient, by letter or telephone, chronologically, with the most recent on top. Documents filed here may include:
- pharmacist's notes,
- copies of letters,
- patient referrals, and
- telephone communications with the patient or health care provider.

Diabetes Care Center
Good Health Pharmacy
411 West Main Street
Stony Brook, VA 23478

February 11, 1998

Jim Belvin, MD
c/o Sarah Mistler's chart
Stony Brook Primary Care Physicians, Inc.
789 East Main Street, Suite #435
Stony Brook, VA 23478

Dear Dr. Belvin:

Thank you again for referring Mrs. Sarah Mistler for diabetes education. The following is a summary of my findings:

CURRENT MEDICATIONS:

Metformin	500 mg PO tid
Hydrochlorothiazide	50 mg 1 PO qAM
Cholestyramine	4 g packet PO tid
Enteric coated aspirin	325 mg qd
Acetaminophen	500 mg 1–2 tabs PO prn headache
Ibuprofen	200 mg 2 tabs PO prn headache
Valerian (unk. strength)	1 cap PO qhs

Objective Monitoring:

1/13/98

Random blood glucose	210 mg/dl
Total Cholesterol	250 mg/dl
HgbA$_{1c}$	10%
Pulse	72 bpm, reg
Blood Pressure-1	158/96
(6 hr post med, rt arm)	
Blood Pressure-2	160/96
(6 hr post med, lt arm)	
Weight	174 lb

2/10/98

Fasting Blood Sugar	225 mg/dl
Fasting Lipid Profile	
Total Cholesterol	248 mg/dl
LDL	165
HDL	40
Triglycerides	215
Pulse	76 bpm, reg
Blood Pressure-1	158/92
(24 hr post med, left)	
Blood Pressure-2	156/94
(24 hr post med, left)	
Weight	173 lb

She was instructed on a glucose meter (AccuCheck Easy) and has been using fairly consistently. Her home monitoring results have been as follows: Average Fasting value = 223 (210–240).

Figure 6. Example letter

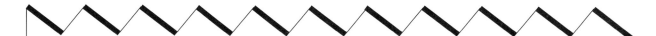

In reviewing Mrs. Mistler's medication profile, discussing her medications with her, and by the above objective values, several issues are raised:

1. She has only beeen taking the Questran 2 times per day. She finds it impossible to take the middle-of-the-day dose. She would like to try something once a day because she thinks she would be able to consistently take this. An HMG CoA reductase inhibitor, such as lovastatin 10 mg qd, would fit this need. Her insurance will cover any of the agents.

2. Although she knows she should be following a diabetic, low-salt, low-fat diet, she has not been. We discussed diet and she has agreed to work on several areas. Although this will likely benefit her disease control, she may need more antidiabetic medication (either an increased dose of metformin or the addition of another medication such as troglitazone). She does very well taking her metformin.

3. Hydrochlorothiazide does not appear to be controlling her blood pressure and may exacerbate her glucose control. An ACE inhibitor, such as enalapril 10 mg qd, may be a good choice for controlling her blood pressure while providing benefits for her diabetes. Again, her insurance covers all of the agents.

4. If there are particular lipid, glucose, hemoglobin A_{1c}, and blood pressure goals you would like her to reach, please convey those to her or me.

5. Since exercise would benefit all her conditions, is Mrs. Mistler a candidate for exercise? Should she have any restrictions on her exercise?

I hope this information is useful. I look forward to continuing to work with you to help Mrs. Mistler reach her medication goals. If you have any comments or questions please call me.

Sincerely,

Susanne Webster

Susanne Webster, R.Ph.

Figure 6. Example letter (continued)

Telephone Contact

Date: April 10, 1998
Time: 9:23 a.m.
With: Dr. Jim Belvin
Re: Sarah Mistler; possible adverse event

Discussion:

Sarah Mistler complained of "little red spots" all over her body. Only change in regimen is that she recently started taking lovastatin for control of hypercholesterolemia. The reaction appeared after 3 days of taking lovastatin. She has not taken it in the past and reports no other medication allergies.

Action taken:

Dr. Belvin wants to see Mrs. Mistler this afternoon. Appointment was scheduled for her. Instructed patient not to take any more lovastatin until seen by Dr. Belvin.

Susanne Webster

Susanne Webster, R.Ph.

Figure 7. Example Telephone Contact Form

This filing procedure will allow you to quickly access the most recent patient visit and review the most recent communications first.

Maintaining Records

Once the organization and location of patient information in the record are established, institute procedures to maintain the patient record, such as:
- filing records alphabetically by the patient's last name,
- maintaining patient confidentiality, and
- storing and maintaining records in a secure location with restricted access.

As a rule, patient records should remain in the care office. In the rare case it is necessary to remove the record, establish a system to keep track of who has the record, when it was removed and returned, and for what purpose.

Creating a Filing System

To facilitate the filing process, you can classify patient records based on patient status. Consider using two levels of activity to define patient status: active or closed. This distinction prevents you from searching through records for patients who are no longer being seen when trying to find a current patient's record.

The patient's file can be considered closed if you expect there will be no future activity. For example, if the patient has not been seen in 6–12 months and has had no clinical interaction that resulted in the generation of a pharmacist's note, the record should be filed as closed. It is advisable to keep closed records for an indefinite period in the event a patient wishes to be seen and for liability reasons. Records are placed in closed status if the patient dies or moves out of the area.

Once status definitions are established, designate appropriate file drawer space to store patient records. Clearly identify each section. File all patient records according to their status first and then alphabetically by the patient's last name.

Summary

Documentation is important for facilitating interactions with patients, continuity of care, reimbursement for services, and legal protection. Many items about patient care must be documented, including patient information gathered, therapy assessments, care plans, monitoring, patient interactions, and communications about the patient. Documentation must be done in an organized and easily retrievable manner.

References

1. American Society of Health-System Pharmacists (ASHP). *Ambulatory Care Clinical Skills: Core Module.* Bethesda, MD: ASHP; 1998. Unit 8, Creating an organized system for assessment of patient problems. p. 149–59.

2. American Society of Health-System Pharmacists (ASHP). *Ambulatory Care Clinical Skills: Core Module.* Bethesda, MD: ASHP; 1998. Unit 7, Recording an ambulatory care pharmacists care plan. p. 133–48.

Self-Study Questions

Objective

Describe elements of a documentation system.

1. Which of the following is an example of a form used to track a patient's subjective and objective data?

    A. Ambulatory Therapy Assessment Worksheet (ATAW)
    B. Ambulatory Monitoring Worksheet (AMW)
    C. Ambulatory Pharmacist's Care Plan (APCP)
    D. Pharmacist's Patient Database Form

2. Explain the rationale for using a systematic documentation system.

3. Describe the role of the Ambulatory Pharmacist's Care Plan (APCP).

Objective

Explain the documentation process, including the use of the SOAP note.

4. Why is it important to complete pharmacist notes in a timely manner?

5. Which of the following best explains why use of the SOAP note is recommended.

    A. The SOAP note is recognized by most health professionals and ensures consistency of information gathered.
    B. The variability of the SOAP format can accommodate the style of each health care professional.
    C. The standardized format decreases the amount of time needed for documentation.
    D. The SOAP format has proved helpful in defending health care providers against claims of medical malpractice.

6. Which of the following is an example of objective information?

    A. results of self-monitoring procedures
    B. reported adherence to medication regimen
    C. reported adverse effects
    D. results of diagnostic procedures

7. Describe the purpose of the assessment and plan sections of a SOAP note.

Objective

Describe the importance of communicating with other health care providers and list methods of communication.

8. Why is it important to communicate information to the patient's other health care providers?

9. Which of the following may be used to communicate with the other health care providers?

    A. letters
    B. pharmacist's notes
    C. telephone conversations
    D. all of the above

Objective

Describe methods to organize and maintain patient records.

10. Explain why a back-up system is needed for an electronic patient record system.

11. A patient's file can be considered closed when:

    A. the patient has not been seen in more than 2 months.
    B. the patient has moved out of the area.
    C. the patient fails to keep three consecutive appointments.
    D. the pharmacy is unable to receive reimbursement for providing cognitive services.

Self-Study Answers

1. B

2. The use of a systematic system provides information in an organized manner that allows for easy retrieval by the pharmacist or other individual providing care. It also allows the pharmacist to track the patient's progress and identify trends and changes in the patient's status.

3. The APCP documents the strategy for patient care; allows for systematic evaluation of pharmacotherapeutic and related health care problems, avoiding the potential to overlook problems; provides a detailed plan or road map for care; and serves as a communication tool between pharmacists providing care.

4. It is important to complete documentation during or shortly after a patient visit because a delay may result in forgetting to include relevant information or confusing information for another patient.

5. A

6. D

7. The assessment section is the assessment of the patient based on the objective and subjective data obtained. The assessment serves as the basis of the plan for addressing patient problems. The plan includes recommendations for correcting the problems identified by the assessment and describes procedures for follow-up.

8. Communication is important to provide other health care providers information about the patient's medication use and progress toward goals. It also fosters the development of professional relationships among providers and establishes the pharmacist as an important member of the care team, whose input can increase the probability of reaching the desired outcomes.

9. D

10. A back-up system is needed in case there is a problem accessing the electronic files (e.g., the computer system is down or files are inadvertently deleted).

11. B

Screening Services

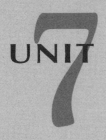

Screening programs can be beneficial to you and your patients. Screening programs provide a public service, serve as a marketing tool for other services you offer, and provide a revenue source (i.e., payment for services). They are used to identify potential health concerns for your customers and thereby allow you to identify potential clients for your other services. By identifying potential health problems, health cost savings can ultimately be realized for the patient by preventing disease progression or hospitalization.

There are several ways to offer screening programs: hire a company that specializes in screening programs to provide the service, partner with a hospital or nursing agency to provide the service, or conduct your own screenings. The method you choose will depend on the cost of the machinery and materials for screening, legal requirements in your state, and your goals in conducting screenings. For example, imagine that you offer a diabetes management program. In this case, one goal of offering screenings may be to attract new patients into the program. Because glucose meters and supplies are relatively inexpensive and your state allows pharmacists to perform laboratory testing, you would offer self-conducted screenings. On the other hand, the machines for bone density screenings for osteoporosis are expensive and many states require a radiology technician perform the testing with machines that use X-ray technology. Your goal in offering bone density screenings may be to provide a public service and generate income. In this case, you may choose to use a screening company. The discussion in this unit will focus on the issues related to self-conducted programs, but many of the issues also apply to other ways of conducting programs.

Unit Objectives

After you successfully complete this unit, you will be able to:
- discuss the types of screening programs that can be provided in an ambulatory patient care service, and
- explain important considerations in planning, advertising, and performing screening tests.

Unit Organization

Unit 7 begins with a description of the types of screening programs that can be conducted in an ambulatory patient care service. Next, a step-by-step process for providing scheduled screening services, including determining tests to provide, screening schedules, testing fees, advertising needs, and required personnel and supplies, is discussed. The need to establish a referral system for patients requiring follow-up is also presented. Test administration and supporting documentation are then explored. The unit concludes with a brief discussion of screening walk-in and existing patients.

Types of Screening Programs

Screenings can be set up in a number of different ways:
- screening days,
- walk-in screenings, or
- screening current patients seen in your practice for undiagnosed conditions.

Screening days are times set aside for screening purposes. Walk-in screening is offering screening at any time without appointments. If you are currently providing a specialty service, such as diabetes care, you can screen your patients with diabetes for hypertension or high cholesterol during your patient interactions.

Advertising Screenings

For all types of screenings, you need to do some marketing to attract patients to the service. Marketing strategies include in-house signage, printed materials, direct mail, and personal communication. You can give patients printed materials about your screening services during their visit to your practice setting. Direct mailings by zip codes are an effective and relatively inexpensive way to promote screenings. Direct communication between the pharmacist and patient is usually the most effective way of marketing value-added pharmacy services.

Establishing a Fee Schedule

You need to establish a fee schedule for your screening services. Fees should include the cost of the test, the cost of associated supplies and services used to conduct the test, and the cost of your time to administer the program. Determine the going rate for these tests in your area and incorporate this information with the actual cost of conducting tests to set your prices. Once fees are established, devise a way to make this information readily available to potential patients. The screening fees could be printed and placed in public view on a sign or flyer.

Screening Days

Screening days can be used to promote your patient care services, provide a value-added service, and serve as a collaborative health-screening effort between you and local hospitals, community health groups (American Diabetes Association, American Heart Association, etc.), or local physician groups. The following are suggestions for establishing and implementing a screening day.

Select the Type of Screening to Be Conducted

Total cholesterol, blood pressure, and blood glucose are commonly performed screening tests. Bone density testing for osteoporosis is a relatively new screening test. **Table 1** lists some advantages and disadvantages of selected screening tests. **Table 2** lists guidelines for screening for high cholesterol, hypertension, diabetes, and osteoporosis.

Which tests you choose to offer will depend on legal requirements for testing within your state, costs of machines and supplies, and competition within your area. See unit 3, Establishing a Laboratory, for information on legal issues related to laboratory testing.

Determine Personnel Requirements

The number of dedicated staff needed for a screening day will depend on the number of tests you will be offering, the time needed to perform each test, and your expected volume. At least one pharmacist will be needed to perform the screenings, and one staff member to process patients and distribute screening related forms. Both duties may be able to be performed by the pharmacist if patient volume is low.

Establish a Date and Time for the Screening Day

Select a day when there will be an adequate number of staff members available. Select a day of the week and time that will elicit the largest patient response. Saturday morning and mid-afternoon are good time periods because patients usually have fewer work conflicts.

Table 1. Advantages and Disadvantages of Selected Screening Tests

Screening	Advantages	Disadvantages
Blood pressure	Inexpensive to perform	Blood pressure screenings are usually accessible to most patient populations and may not elicit a large patient response
Blood glucose	Inexpensive to perform Ability to collaborate with meter manufacturers	Time and content of last meal can affect screening results and interpretation
Total cholesterol	No fasting required Elicits good patient response	More costly to perform than blood pressure or blood glucose
Bone mineral density (for osteoporosis)	May be a new service not offered routinely in your community Requires no patient preparation Screening companies can reduce cost to individual hosting event and provide complete screening service, including personnel and camera-ready advertising	Regulations on who may perform test and whether a doctor's order is required vary by state Cost of testing equipment

Table 2. Screening Recommendations

Diabetes[a] All symptomatic, undiagnosed individuals 45 years or older
If values are normal, repeat every 3 years
Test at younger age or more frequent intervals in individuals who:
- are obese ($\geq$120% of desirable body weight or BMI $\geq$27 kg/m²)
- have a first-degree relative with diabetes
- are members of a high-risk ethnic population (e.g., African-American, Hispanic, Native American)
- have delivered a baby weighing >9 lb or have been diagnosed with gestational diabetes mellitus
- are hypertensive ($\geq$140/90)
- have an HDL cholesterol level $\leq$ 35 mg/dl and/or a triglyceride level $\geq$ 250 mg/dl
- had impaired glucose tolerance (fasting glucose between 110 mg/dl and 126 mg/dl) on a previous test

Cholesterol[b, c] NCEP: Screen all persons aged 20 years and older every 5 years
ACP: Screen men 35–65 and women 45–60 if desired but not considered mandatory.
Screening in men and women between 65–75 years old is neither recommended nor discouraged
Screening is not recommended for men and women older than 75.
Only screen young adults (men <35 and women <45) if there is evidence of familial lipid disease or at least two other cardiac risk factors.
Retest every 5 years if the initial level is close to a treatment threshold

Hypertension[d, e] Screen all adults any time they seek medical care

Osteoporosis[f] Bone mineral density screening can be performed for risk assessment in perimenopausal or postmenopausal women who are concerned about osteoporosis and willing to accept available interventions and in women at high risk for osteoporosis (family history, long-term glucocorticoid therapy, hyperparathyroidism, etc.)

BMI, body mass index; HDL, high-density lipoprotein.

[a] Report of the expert committee on the diagnosis and classification of diabetes mellitus. *Diabetes Care* 1997;20:1183–97.

[b] American College of Physicians. Guidelines for using serum cholesterol, high density lipoprotein cholesterol, and triglyceride levels as screening tests for preventing coronary heart disease in adults. *Ann Intern Med* 1996;124:515–7.

[c] Summary of the second report of the National Cholesterol Education Program (NCEP) expert panel on detection, evaluation, and treatment of high blood cholesterol in adults (adult treatment panel II). *JAMA* 1993;269:3015–23.

[d] Littenberg B. A practice guideline revisited: screening for hypertension. *Ann Intern Med* 1995;122:937–9.

[e] Littenberg B, Garber AM, Sox HC. Screening for hypertension. *Ann Intern Med* 1990;112:192–202.

[f] American Association of Clinical Endocrinologists. AACE Clinical Practice Guidelines for the Prevention and Treatment of Postmenopausal Osteoporosis. *Endocr Pract* 1996;2:155–71.

Establish a Duration for Screenings

A 4- to 6-hour time slot is usually adequate. The goal is to maximize productivity during the designated time slot while minimizing downtime.

Advertise

Begin advertising 2–3 weeks before the screening day. Be sure to have promotional materials for your other services on hand during the screenings so that you can market these as well. An example of an advertisement for a screening is in **Figure 1**.

Obtain Necessary Supplies

Make sure you have an adequate amount of test reagents on hand before the screening day. It is often hard to predict the number of patients that will show up for a screening, making it difficult to order an accurate amount of supplies. As a general rule, the greater your advertising effort, the greater the number of patients who will participate.

Establish a Referral Procedure

You must make a reasonable effort to ensure that patients with an abnormal result follow up with a physician. Although one abnormal result does not usually prompt a diagnosis, the result should be evaluated by the patient's physician and repeated if necessary. Options for referral and follow-up include providing the screening results to patients with instruction to follow up with their physician and/or sending the results directly to the physician. For patients without a physician, you may wish to have information available about local physician practices so patients can schedule an appointment. For patients who may not be able to afford to see a physician, you should have information on low-cost medical care services, if available, in your community.

Perform Screenings

A procedure for screening patients is outlined in **Table 3**. A screening questionnaire is included as **Figure 2** and in **Appendix 1**. This questionnaire or something similar is used to evaluate patients for the appropriateness of screening tests and to assist in the interpretation of the results. In addition to reviewing patients' medical histories with a questionnaire, you should consider having patients sign liability waiver forms. An example liability waiver form is included as **Figure 3**. This form releases you from liability related to obtaining a blood sample and advises patients to consult their physician about the results. Example screening result forms for selected tests are included as **Figures 4** through **7**. These forms provide a written interpretation of the results for the patient. Blank liability and screening result forms are included in **Appendix 1**.

You should document the results of all screenings and your actions based on the results. Maintain a screening file containing screening questionnaire, liability waiver form, and documentation of results and the interaction with each patient.

Evaluate Results

After the screening day, evaluate how many screenings were performed, patient comments, and staff thoughts. Look for areas to improve on for future screening days.

Table 3. Suggested Screening Procedure

- Determine which tests the patient is requesting.
- Inform patient of the fee associated with the screening.
- Provide the patient with instructions on testing procedure if appropriate.
- Schedule an appointment, if needed, to perform the screening at the appropriate time.
- Have the patient sign a Liability Waiver Form.
- Ask the patient to complete a Patient Screening Questionnaire.
- Review the questionnaire with the patient and determine risk factor analysis, if appropriate.
- Explain test(s) and procedure(s) to the patient. Make sure the patient understands you are screening and not diagnosing.
- Perform requested test(s).
- Discuss result(s) with the patient.
- Provide the patient with a written copy of the results.
- If appropriate, refer the patient to his/her physician.
- Collect payment.
- Document patient screening results and your actions based on the results.
- File all documentation related to the screening (questionnaire, waiver form, any notes).

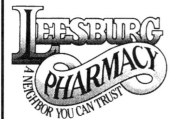 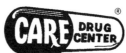
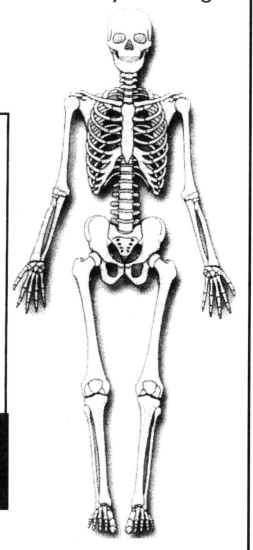
Figure 1. Advertisement for screening

Patient Screening Questionnaire

I. Type of Screening

Please put a check (✓) next to the screening tests listed below that you wish to have performed:

- ✓ blood glucose
- ✓ total cholesterol
- ✓ HDL cholesterol
- _____ total cholesterol/HDL cholesterol ratio
- ✓ lipid profile
- ✓ blood pressure

II. Patient Information

Date: __1-13-98__

Name: __Sarah Mistler__

Address: __Rt.1 Box 485__
__Stony Brook, VA 23478__

Home Phone: __200-0012__

Office Phone: __--__

Date of Birth: __1-4-40__   Age: __58__

Name of Health Insurer: __Blue Cross, Blue Shield__

Health Ins. Card # __3561789592__

Social Security #: __123-45-6789__

Primary Care Physician's Name: __Dr. Jim Belvin__

Phone: __555-0001__

Specialist Physician's Name: __--__

Phone: __--__

Date and time of last food or beverage __7pm 1-12-98__

III. Medical History

Please put a check (✓) next to the statements that are true:

- ✓ I have high blood pressure.
- ✓ I take medication for high blood pressure.
- ✓ I have diabetes.
- ✓ I take medication for diabetes.
- ✓ I have high cholesterol.
- ✓ I take medication for high cholesterol.
- _____ I have had a stroke.
- _____ I have had heart bypass surgery
- _____ I have had a heart attack.

IV. Heart Disease Risk Factors

Please put a check (✓) next to the statements which are true:

- ✓ I have high blood pressure.
- ✓ I have diabetes.
- ✓ I smoke cigarettes.
- _____ I am a male over the age of 45.
- ✓ I am a female over the age of 55.
- _____ I am a female less than 55 years old, I have had my ovaries removed, and I am not taking estrogen therapy.
- ✓ My father or brother died of a heart attack before age 55.
- _____ My mother or sister died of a heart attack before age 65.
- _____ I have had chest pain (angina).
- _____ I have had heart bypass surgery.

I certify to the best of my knowledge the above information is true.

__Sarah Mistler__
(signature)

Figure 2. Patient Screening Questionnaire

LIABILITY WAIVER

I hereby consent to have blood samples drawn for the purpose of screening. I understand that there may be some discomfort, bruising, bleeding, or swelling at the puncture site and surrounding tissue, and that it may become infected. If signs of infection are seen (redness, swelling, warmth, pain, or pus), I will seek medical care.

I hereby release **Good Health Pharmacy**, their affiliates, directors, officers, employees, successors, and assigns from any and all liability arising from or in any way connected with this blood drawing for my measurements or from the data derived therefrom. I understand that:

I should not participate in this test if I suffer from any bleeding disorder or similar condition.

The data derived from this test are to be considered preliminary only and must be confirmed with additional tests. We advise that you review the results of this test with your physician.

Date: **1-13-98**

Name: **Sarah Mistler**

Signature: **Sarah Mistler**

Figure 3. Liability Waiver Form

DIABETES SCREENING RESULTS

Diabetes is a condition in which the body cannot use sugar (also referred to as glucose) properly. There are about 14 million people with diabetes in the United States. Half of them have not yet been diagnosed. It is important to diagnose diabetes early. Early detection and treatment may limit some of the long-term complications of diabetes. These include vision loss, kidney disease, heart disease, nerve damage, and damage to the blood vessels in the legs, feet, and hands.

Your chance of developing diabetes is greater if you:
- are overweight
- have a family history of diabetes
- are a woman who delivered babies weighing over 9 pounds or had diabetes during pregnancy
- are African American
- are Hispanic
- are a Native American

Many symptoms can occur if a patient has diabetes. Each patient will have different symptoms. Some patients have severe symptoms while others have no symptoms at all. Some symptoms of diabetes include:
- more frequent urination
- increased thirst
- tiredness
- weakness
- dizziness
- increased hunger
- slow wound healing
- more frequent infections

In a person without diabetes the blood glucose level is normally 60–126 mg/dl (milligrams of glucose in each deciliter of blood). Results above 126 mg/dl are considered high and measurements below 60 mg/dl are considered low.

A single high reading does not mean you have diabetes, but you should see your doctor for further evaluation.

Your blood glucose is: **210 mg/dl**

Date: **1-13-98**

Time: **10 A.M.**

Date last food or beverage was consumed:
1-12-98

Time last food or beverage was consumed:
7 p.m.

Figure 4. Diabetes Screening Results Form

BLOOD PRESSURE SCREENING RESULTS

The heart is a muscle that pumps blood through the blood vessels in the body. When the heart beats, it squeezes blood into the blood vessels and creates pressure in them. This pressure is needed to circulate blood through the entire body. The heart beats 60–100 times each minute and rests between each beat.

Blood pressure is highest when the heart beats and lowest when the heart rests. Therefore, a patient really has two levels of blood pressure: an upper one when the heart is beating and a lower one when the heart is resting. The higher pressure is called the systolic pressure. The lower pressure is referred to as the diastolic pressure. The systolic blood pressure is important because it tells the maximum amount of pressure placed on the blood vessels. The diastolic pressure tells the minimum amount of pressure placed on the blood vessels.

Both the diastolic and systolic levels are recorded when your blood pressure is measured. For example, if your blood pressure reading is recorded as 110/85 (110 over 85), the top number (110) is the systolic pressure and the bottom number (85) is the diastolic pressure. Blood pressure is measured in the units "mmHg" (millimeters of mercury).

When someone's blood pressure is higher than the desirable range, they have hypertension. *Hyper* means high and *tension* refers to pressure. For most adults a blood pressure reading above 140/90 mmHg is considered higher than the desirable range. Adults who have diabetes or kidney damage have a lower desirable range.

In about 90% of people with hypertension, the cause is unknown. Several factors seem to increase the risk for developing hypertension. These include heredity; male gender; older age; black race; obesity; sensitivity to sodium; heavy alcohol consumption; the use of certain medications such as decongestants, nonsteroidal anti-inflammatory agents, and products containing sodium; smoking; and an inactive lifestyle.

Over 60 million Americans have hypertension. In general, hypertension has no symptoms, but if untreated it can lead to serious complications, such as stroke, heart attacks, and heart failure. Some patients may complain of headache or changes in vision such as blurred vision, but most people are not aware they have hypertension until they have their blood pressure measured.

A single high reading does not mean you have hypertension, but you should see your doctor for further evaluation.

Your blood pressure today is: **158/96 mmHg**

Date: **1-13-98**

Time: **10 A.M.**

Figure 5. Blood Pressure Screening Results Form

CHOLESTEROL SCREENING RESULTS

Cholesterol is a fat-like substance found in all your body's cells. Cholesterol is used to make cell membranes and certain hormones in your body. Problems may occur when you have too much cholesterol.

Cholesterol comes from two sources. It is produced normally in your body and also comes from certain foods in your diet. Cholesterol travels throughout the body to where it is needed. Because cholesterol is made up of fat, it cannot travel through the blood by itself (fat cannot mix with water). Instead it must be transported to and from cells by special carriers called lipoproteins. There are several types of lipoproteins, but the ones we are most concerned about are low-density lipoprotein (LDL) and high-density lipoprotein (HDL).

LDL is called "bad" cholesterol because it sticks to the inside wall of blood vessels, increasing the chance of developing coronary heart disease. HDL cholesterol, or "good" cholesterol, rescues LDL that is stuck on the blood vessel wall and returns it to the liver.

Triglycerides are a type of fat found in lipoproteins. Various lipoproteins contain different amounts of triglycerides. The triglyceride level in the blood is highest right after eating a meal containing fat.

If your cholesterol level is too high, LDL cholesterol will deposit in the blood vessels that supply the heart muscle with blood and oxygen and narrow the blood vessels. This is referred to as coronary artery disease. Eventually the blood vessels narrow so much that the blood supply is decreased. When the blood supply decreases, the heart muscle does not receive enough oxygen and is damaged. A heart attack occurs when there is damage to the heart muscle.

In general, total blood cholesterol should be less than 200 mg/dl (milligrams of cholesterol per deciliter of blood). If the total cholesterol is above 200 mg/dl, it is considered too high.

A single high reading does not mean you have high cholesterol, but you should see your doctor for further evaluation. You may need to have another test of your cholesterol which tells you how much "good" and "bad" cholesterol you have in your blood. This test is called a lipid profile.

Your total cholesterol is: __250 mg/dl__

Date: ___1-13-98___

Time: ___10 A.M.___

Date last food or beverage was consumed: ___1-12-98___

Time last food or beverage was consumed: ___7 P.M.___

Figure 6. Cholesterol Screening Results Form

CHOLESTEROL SCREENING RESULTS (FOR FULL LIPID PROFILE)

Cholesterol is a fat-like substance found in all your body's cells. Cholesterol is used to make cell membranes and certain hormones in your body. Problems may occur when you have too much cholesterol.

Cholesterol comes from two sources. It is produced normally in your body and also comes from certain foods in your diet. Cholesterol travels throughout the body to where it is needed. Because cholesterol is made up of fat, it cannot travel through the blood by itself (fat cannot mix with water). Instead it must be transported to and from cells by special carriers called lipoproteins. There are several types of lipoproteins, but the ones we are most concerned about are low-density lipoprotein (LDL) and high-density lipoprotein (HDL).

LDL is called "bad" cholesterol because it sticks to the inside wall of blood vessels, increasing the chance of developing coronary heart disease. HDL cholesterol, or "good" cholesterol, rescues LDL that is stuck on the blood vessel wall and returns it to the liver.

Triglycerides are a type of fat found in lipoproteins. Various lipoproteins contain different amounts of triglycerides. The triglyceride level in the blood is highest right after eating a meal containing fat.

If your cholesterol level is too high, LDL cholesterol will deposit in the blood vessels that supply the heart muscle with blood and oxygen and narrow the blood vessels. This is referred to as coronary artery disease. Eventually the blood vessels narrow so much that the blood supply is decreased. When the blood supply decreases, the heart muscle does not receive enough oxygen and is damaged. A heart attack occurs when there is damage to the heart muscle.

In general, total blood cholesterol should be less than 200 mg/dl (milligrams of cholesterol per deciliter of blood). If the total cholesterol is above 200 mg/dl, it is considered too high.

The triglyceride level in the blood should be less than 250 mg/dl.

The HDL cholesterol level should be more than 35 mg/dl.

The recommended goal for LDL cholesterol depends on two criteria. The first is the presence of coronary artery disease and the second is the number of coronary heart disease risk factors.

Risk factors for coronary heart disease are conditions that increase a person's chance of developing coronary heart disease. These risk factors include:

- being a male over the age of 45
- being a female over the age of 55 OR being a female under the age of 55 who is not taking hormone replacement therapy after having both ovaries removed.
- having a male sibling or parent who died of a heart attack or had a heart attack before age 55
- having a female parent or sibling who died of a heart attack or had a heart attack before age 65
- smoking cigarettes
- having high blood pressure
- having diabetes
- having a low HDL cholesterol (less than 35 mg/dl [milligrams of HDL cholesterol in each deciliter of blood])

Figure 7. Cholesterol Screening Results (for Full Lipid Profile) Form

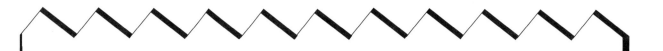

If you have coronary heart disease, your LDL cholesterol should be less than 100 mg/dl.

If you do not have coronary artery disease but have two or more risk factors for coronary heart disease, your LDL cholesterol should be less than 130 mg/dl.

If you do not have coronary heart disease and have less than two risk factors for coronary heart disease, your LDL cholesterol should be less than 160 mg/dl.

A single high reading does not mean you have high cholesterol, but you should see your doctor for further evaluation.

Your total cholesterol is: **248 mg/dl**

Your HDL cholesterol is: **40 mg/dl**

Your LDL cholesterol is: **165 mg/dl**

Your triglycerides are: **215 mg/dl**

Date: **2-10-98**

Time: **10 A.M.**

Date last food or beverage was consumed: **2-9-98**

Time last food or beverage was consumed: **7 p.m.**

Figure 7. Cholesterol Screening Results (for Full Lipid Profile) Form (continued)

At your appointment on __1-13-98__, we will measure your fasting blood glucose level. A fasting measurement is the most consistent blood glucose level. If you are taking medicine for diabetes, a fasting level helps us evaluate how well your medicine works overnight. Please observe the following directions to ensure the results are accurate:

THE DAY BEFORE THE TEST

After __7 P.M.__, (time) do not eat or drink anything except water.

THE DAY OF THE TEST

Do not eat or drink anything except water until after the test is performed.

DO NOT take your diabetes medication (oral agent and/or insulin) until after the test is performed.

Take all other medications as directed.

If you have any questions, please contact your pharmacist at __200-0044__.

Figure 8. Instructions for fasting blood glucose screening

At your appointment on __2-10-98__, we will measure your fasting lipid profile. This test will allow us to measure your LDL cholesterol, HDL cholesterol, triglycerides, and total cholesterol level. Because some of these values are affected by food, it is important that you observe the following directions to be sure the results are accurate:

THE DAY BEFORE THE TEST

After __9 P.M.__, (time) do not eat or drink anything except water.

THE DAY OF THE TEST

Do not eat or drink anything except water until after the test is performed.

Take all of your medications as usual.

If you have any questions, please contact your pharmacist at __200-0044__.

Figure 9. Instructions for fasting lipid profile

At your appointment on _____1-13-98_____,
we will measure your blood pressure. Please
observe the following directions to be sure
the results are accurate:

THE DAY OF THE TEST

Take all of your medications as directed,
including your blood pressure medication.

Wear clothing that does not limit the
blood flow in the arms when the blood pressure
measurement is performed. (Restrictive
clothing can falsely elevate the blood pressure).

Arrive at least 10 minutes early so that
you can be seated comfortably and rest before
the measurement. (Physical activity and
stress can falsely elevate the blood pressure).

30 MINUTES BEFORE THE APPOINTMENT

1. Do not drink beverages that contain
   caffeine (such as coffee, tea, or soft
   drinks) 30 minutes before the appointment. (Caffeine can falsely
   elevate blood pressure.)

2. Do not use tobacco products 30
   minutes before the appointment. This
   includes cigarettes, cigars, and
   chewing tobacco. (Nicotine can
   falsely elevate blood pressure.)

If you have any questions, please contact
your pharmacist at ___200-0044___.

Figure 10. Instructions for blood pressure screening

Walk-In Screenings

You can also offer screenings on a walk-in basis
during your usual hours of operation. Promote walk-
ins with a sign that can be posted when a pharmacist
is available to perform screenings. Walk-in screenings are an excellent way to generate interest in and
promote your other services.

One risk of offering service on a walk-in basis is
that the pharmacist may not always be available
when a patient requests a test. If the pharmacist is
busy and the patient is unable to wait, use an
appointment system to schedule the patient for the
screening at a mutually agreeable time. If you are
offering screening tests that require a period of
fasting or other special instructions (e.g., fasting
lipid profile), you may wish to schedule patients for
appointments and provide them with written
instructions on how to prepare for the test. Examples
of written instructions for selected tests are given in
Figures 8 through **10**. Blank forms are included in
Appendix 1.

Screening Existing Patients

To identify potentially undiagnosed conditions, you
can screen patients you currently see in your patient
care practice as appropriate based on the national
guidelines for screenings, unless they have had the
testing done elsewhere (**Table 2**).

Summary

A screening program, whether targeted at existing
patients or walk-ins or held as one-time events, can
provide many benefits for the pharmacist. These
programs are easy to set up and provide not only a
public service but also marketing and financial
rewards for the pharmacist.

Self-Study Questions

Objective

Discuss the types of screening programs that can be provided in an ambulatory patient care service.

1. List the three types of screening services that are possible in an ambulatory patient care service.

2. Describe the potential advantages and disadvantages of providing walk-in screening services.

Objective

Explain important considerations in planning, advertising, and performing screening tests.

3. Which of the following is considered the most effective marketing campaign for screening services?

    A. store signs
    B. flyers
    C. direct mailings
    D. direct patient communication

4. The determination of the test fee is best described by which of the following statements?

    A. The charge should be based on what the patient can afford to pay for the test.
    B. The charge should equal the reimbursement given by the patient's insurance.
    C. The charge should include the cost of testing supplies plus administrative costs.
    D. The charge should include the cost of the testing supplies, administrative costs, and a consideration of the average test charge in the geographic area.

5. Describe factors important to consider when selecting the type of screening tests to offer.

6. Explain the importance of establishing a referral mechanism.

7. Useful forms for conducting screening services include all of the following *except*:

    A. care plans.
    B. liability waiver forms.
    C. screening questionnaires.
    D. pretest instructions.

Self-Study Answers

1. Screening services can be provided for scheduled, walk-in, or existing patients with undiagnosed conditions.

2. Walk-in testing is an inexpensive way to promote program services that allows you decrease testing cost by only providing services as staffing permits. Disadvantages include that the pharmacist may not be available for testing when the patient arrives. Walk-in testing also precludes certain tests, such as those that require a period of fasting.

3. D

4. D

5. The selection of screening tests to be offered should consider patient needs, including current and targeted patient populations; the cost of tests; state legal requirements; and the testing services offered by other providers in your area.

6. It is the responsibility of the ambulatory patient care service to refer and encourage patients with abnormal test results to seek follow-up treatments. The service should communicate with a patient's physician and have information available for patients who do not have, or cannot afford, physician services.

7. A

Marketing

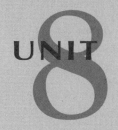

Marketing is selling a product or service. Successful programs require effective, ongoing marketing. It is challenging to market pharmaceutical care services because many patients and health care providers are not familiar with the concept. It is difficult to sell a service people are not familiar with or have not experienced. To introduce people to this new concept, you focus on why they should participate (i.e., the benefits to them) and how the concept works.

Who you market to will depend on your setting. You have to identify who will benefit from and be affected by your services and develop a marketing effort for each group. The purpose of this unit is to help you identify who to market your services to and the types of marketing activities you can do.

Unit Objectives

After you successfully complete this unit, you will be able to:
- identify target audiences when marketing your services, and
- describe elements of an effective marketing plan.

Unit Organization

This unit begins with a brief review of setting-specific factors that need to be considered when preparing the marketing plan for your services. Potential target groups for marketing efforts are then defined and effective strategies for marketing to these groups are explored. Next, the need for ongoing marketing efforts is discussed. The unit concludes with an example marketing plan for a health-system pharmacy.

Initial Strategy

Before you begin providing patient care services, you need to take a few steps to develop your marketing plan. The first of these steps was outlined in unit 1. To review, you need to do a global assessment of your setting that includes identifying:
- potential payers for your services and their unmet needs,
- the purpose (goals) of the business,
- the skills and interests of staff,
- competition,

- the services offered by the business,
- the customers of the business (in addition to payers), and
- the realistic financial goals and market potential of the business.

After completing this global assessment, you need to identify the target audiences for your marketing efforts and develop a marketing plan for each audience, with a timeline for implementation.

Identify Your Audience

In general, you will market to two primary groups: someone to pay for your services (i.e., the potential payers you identified earlier) and the users of the service who must participate for you to get paid (i.e., patients or physicians, if a referral is necessary).

A primary target for your marketing efforts should be whomever would have to pay for the consequences of drug-related morbidity, because that person should willingly pay to prevent these consequences.[1] Identify who is ultimately at risk for the costs of patient care you can affect (i.e., hospitalizations, emergency room visits, medications, and treatment of adverse effects). This party may be the patient, employer, third-party payer (i.e., insurance company, HMO, or preferred provider organization), physician group (if reimbursed a set fee to provide all care to a patient [i.e., capitation]), health care system, hospital (if capitated), or the government. For example, in a hospital-based diabetes clinic where the hospital is capitated for all hospitalization costs for a group of diabetes patients, the potential payer for your services or party at risk is the hospital. Employers who are self-insured or have long-term risks for substantial portions of their employee population may promote to their insurers or plan administrators the inclusion of a pharmacist-provided disease prevention program to reduce health care costs and sick days.

In addition to the party at risk, you need to market to those who will use your services. They may be patients, individual physicians, physician practices, payers, or the management of health care systems and businesses. Identify the users of the service who must participate for you to get paid and whomever else will benefit from or be affected by your services. For example, in the hospital-based diabetes clinic mentioned above, physicians (if referrals to the clinic are necessary), patients (if they are allowed to elect to come to the clinic), and hospital management would all be affected by your services. Therefore, they are your other target audiences. Strategies for marketing to each audience are presented later in this unit.

Target Groups in Specific Settings

HMO

In the HMO setting, you need to market primarily to management and physicians. The HMO or the purchaser of the HMO's services will be the payer for your services in this setting. Because physicians are the users of your services by providing you with patient referrals, you need to market to them rather than directly to patients. Enlist the help of the HMO management and/or senior medical management to market your services to physicians and to identify appropriate patients for your services. Their endorsement will help you succeed.

Clinic/Physician's Office

In a clinic or physician's office setting, the payers for your services will depend on the payment system for the setting. You may need to market to the major insurers of the patient population or to the physician group or hospital, if they are capitated. In a clinic or doctor's office setting, physicians will be the primary users of your services because you will depend on them for referrals. Patients will not likely be a direct target for your efforts.

Community/Retail Setting

Because the community or retail setting is usually not part of a health care system, your marketing efforts must be much broader. Most important, you will have to market to payers, who are, as discussed before, the party at risk for patient care costs. The payers may be insurers, employers, capitated physicians, health care systems, or hospitals. The users of your services will be patients and/or physicians, depending on how patients will access your services (i.e., self- or physician referral). Retail management must also be targets of your marketing, so that they foster an environment that supports patient care services, as discussed in unit 1.

Develop a Marketing Plan

You must have a plan for marketing. Selling is an ongoing process that, to be effective, cannot be done haphazardly. Your plan, which does not have to be elaborate, should specify who you are targeting, how you plan to market to each group, how you plan to follow up on the effectiveness of your efforts, and when you plan to market to each group (i.e., an implementation time line). Some of your marketing efforts will only occur before beginning to provide services, whereas others will be ongoing. For example, you may need to initially sell your idea of a patient care service to management, but marketing to patients and physicians is a more continual process.

In developing your marketing plan, you need to consider what resources are available to you. Consider how much money is available for developing, producing, and distributing materials. Consider whether you have access, either from within your organization or outside, to other people who can develop materials and do the marketing for you. Even with minimal funds and doing the work yourself, you can develop effective marketing materials. For example, you may have a budget of $500 for all your marketing efforts and no inside help for development or distribution. You can choose to spend the money on glossy brochures printed by an outside printer, or you can print brochures yourself using color papers from an office supply store, mail letters to target physicians, and host an open house with refreshments.

An important marketing resource in most settings are supporters and collaborators to help you sell your services. You will usually need to identify a champion for your cause in both management and among important physicians. The physician should be someone who is well respected by colleagues (i.e., is an opinion leader), supports your cause, and is willing to advocate your services to management and other physicians. This will help increase the chance for success. In addition, consider other pharmacists, nurse practitioners and physician's office personnel in the area who can make referrals and help promote your practice.

Recommended Strategies for Specific Groups

Patients

Before marketing to patients, you need to identify which patients you plan to target. Create a list of eligible patients who would benefit from the services you plan to offer. There are several ways to create this list:

- Generate a list from dispensing records based on therapeutic drug class, disease state, third-party payer, or combination of appropriate variables. This method is fairly accurate for asthma, diabetes, and hyperlipidemia patients. Identifying patients with other conditions, such as hypertension, can be more tedious, because antihypertensives can be used to treat multiple medical problems such as edema, congestive heart failure, and arrhythmias.

- Obtain a list of patients selected by the payer of your services. Generally, these will be patients who are high-volume consumers of health care services.
- Offer screening services.

Patient Marketing Strategies

When marketing to patients, it is important to describe why they should participate, so they understand how your services will benefit them. For patients to participate, there needs to be commitment and understanding regarding the potential benefits. In addition, it is important to describe how the program operates, so patients know what to expect. Include information such as the nature of the interaction, expected time commitment, topics addressed, etc.

For example, if you are marketing a monitoring and management program for diabetic patients, you might list the expected benefits using the following presentation:

Our specially trained pharmacist will work closely with you to:

- give you the facts needed to use your medication correctly and point out the signs you should look for to avoid possible problems,
- help you organize your medications for easy use,
- provide you with routine checkpoints of your progress towards your diabetes management goals,
- see that you have the information and support you need to make positive changes in your lifestyle, and
- answer any questions you may have about home glucose monitoring and show you how and when to take blood sugar measurements for the most accurate results.

Here's how the program works:

- You can call ahead for an appointment that fits your schedule.
- In the privacy of our Care Center, our pharmacist will review all medications you're taking and talk to you about how you've been feeling and any changes you may have noticed.
- We may make recommendations that can improve the effects of your prescriptions and help avoid or reduce the side effects that

sometimes occur with diabetes medicines.

- We'll check your blood glucose level with a simple blood sample taken from your finger, give you a copy of the results, and send a copy to your doctor.
- If we should notice anything either in your blood glucose reading or in what you have to say that makes us think a change might be indicated, we'll work with you and your doctor to help you achieve the desired goals.

Marketing efforts directed at patients may include incentives, a program logo and name, signage, direct mailings, brochures, menu of services, face-to-face discussions, and outside advertising. You can also participate in community organizations and offer to give talks to these organizations. Do not expect one marketing tool to single-handedly promote your services to patients. Instead, develop a marketing package that incorporates several tools.

Incentives

An especially effective tool for marketing to patients is the offer of incentives for participation. If you are trying to attract self-pay patients, you might offer free introductory services, coupons for discounts on items related to patients' conditions, or free product samples. Free introductory visits allow potential patients to experience your services firsthand. This will give you an opportunity to talk to patients about the scope and importance of your patient care services. Introductory services can be as simple as a drug utilization review, the development of a medication scheduling plan, or a blood pressure screening.

Payers can also offer incentives to entice patients to participate in your services. Financial rewards for participation, such as reduced prescription co-payments or free self-monitoring supplies, are especially effective.

Program Logo and Name

A program logo and name should be developed with distinctive colors and fonts to allow patients to recognize the patient care services as unique from other products and services. The logo should be printed on all materials associated with the program (signs, brochures, letterhead, envelopes, and medical history forms).

Signage

Signage provides recognition of the patient care services to every patient who reads them. Signage describing the program and its benefits to potential patients should be placed in noticeable locations. An example sign is included in **Figure 1**.

Ask the pharmacist

about our new programs
for people with:

ASTHMA

DIABETES

HIGH BLOOD PRESSURE

HIGH CHOLESTEROL

Figure 1. Example sign

Direct Mailings to Patients

Introductory letters describing the program and its potential benefits can be sent to potential patients. These letters can come directly from you, from the payer of your services, or from the physician referral source, depending on your setting. A sample letter from a pharmacist is included in **Figure 2**.

Marketing Brochures

A marketing brochure describes why your services are beneficial and the operating procedure involved. Brochures can be displayed in racks in prominent places, mailed to potential patients, or given personally to patients. An example marketing brochure is included in **Figure 3**.

Fee Schedule

If you are seeking payment from patients or billing an insurance company, you need to have a printed fee schedule available to explain the cost of your services to patients, because they will be responsible for payment of the full amount or the amount not covered by their insurance.

Pharmacist Marketing

In addition to distributing written marketing materials, you should give a personalized verbal description of your services to the patient. A personalized sales pitch is the *most* successful recruitment tool. Distributing pieces of paper does not convince patients they need patient care services. You need to individualize your marketing effort to explain to patients how and why they will benefit.

Screenings

Screening programs in your pharmacy serve to identify potential health concerns for patients and allow you to provide information about your services. Refer to unit 7, Screening Services, for further information.

Other Methods

There are several methods to advertise to potential patients who may not be targeted by the previously discussed efforts, including newspaper, radio, and television advertisements and promotional events. Work in conjunction with manufacturers to offer promotional events to minimize the cost of advertising your patient care program. For example, offer a meter day where patients can trade in their old glucose meters for the latest model in conjunction with a home glucose meter manufacturer. The manufacturer may be willing to contribute to or cover the cost of advertising the day. During the event, you can promote your patient care services to participants.

Educate Staff

Take time before patient care services are initiated to explain the purpose and operation to your support staff (clerks, technicians, cashiers, managers, etc.). They need to understand that you will be changing your priorities to focus on direct patient care.

Support staff should be able to answer questions from potential patients, including:

- What does this new service involve?
- Why is this program good for me?
- How often will this service be provided and how much time will it take?
- What is the cost?

Some important reminders when explaining patient care services to a patient:

- Make it brief.
- Use terminology the patient understands.
- Be careful not to use words that may offend or stigmatize the patient, such as "disease." Many patients may be offended to have a label placed on them, such as "having a chronic disease" or "having a particular disease."
- Remember that a patient's medical history is confidential. When a patient refers someone to you, be careful not to reveal to that person the diseases or conditions of the patient who referred the person. Use common sense.

Good Health Pharmacy

411 West Main Street   Stony Brook, VA 23478

December 30, 1997

Sarah Mistler
Rte. 1, Box 485
Stony Brook, VA 23478

Dear Sarah,

I am writing to tell you about the Diabetes Care Program we have implemented in Good Health Pharmacy in Stony Brook, VA.

The Diabetes Care Program provides a number of special services for patients who take medications for diabetes. Our goal is to make sure these patients on long-term therapy get the best results possible from their medication through this special program.

As part of this program, I will provide you with the following:
- private consultations to discuss how your medicine is working and any problems or questions;
- regular monitoring of your condition to look for possible side effects and check your progress toward your personal health goals;
- educational material about your condition, the medications you are taking, and how certain activities can help your medications work better; and
- regular reports to your physician so he or she will know how you are doing between physician visits.

We are committed to providing you with the best professional consultation, medical information, and monitoring that is available today. Please stop in to see me at Good Health Pharmacy, or give me a call at 200-0044 to ask any questions. Together with you and your doctor, we can make the best use of your medications, ensuring you have a healthy life.

Sincerely,

SUSANNE WEBSTER

Susanne Webster, R.Ph.

Figure 2. Sample introductory letter to potential patients

Introducing

THE PHARMACY CARE CENTER

for

Diabetic Patients

Now you and your doctor can both be sure your diabetes is being controlled between office visits—with regular mini-checkups right here in our Pharmacy Care Center!

- PRIVATE
- PERSONALIZED
- INFORMATIVE
- CONVENIENT

A complete program of monitoring and professional advice to give you more control over your health!

It Costs So Little to Be Sure, at the PHARMACY CARE CENTER!

We have special pricing for anyone registering for the initial year's program of consultation and monitoring in the **Pharmacy Care Center**. You will receive a full year of blood glucose monitoring—including pharmacy counseling throughout the year. We will measure your blood glucose levels and blood pressure on every visit, and we will monitor other areas as well.

Special combination fees are also available for diabetic patients who have high blood pressure, asthma, and/or high cholesterol. The **Pharmacy Care Center** has programs to help patients with any of these conditions.

For more information, or to schedule an appointment, talk to your pharmacist about the special programs in the **Pharmacy Care Center**. We're here to help you be sure you get your medicine's worth!

Here's how THE PROGRAM WORKS:

- You can call ahead for an appointment that fits your schedule or arrange for a mini-checkup when you come in for a refill. Either way, for best results you should see your pharmacist periodically throughout the year.

- In the privacy of our **Pharmacy Care Center**, our pharmacist will review all medications you're taking and talk to you about how you've been feeling and any changes you may have noticed.

- The pharmacist may also make recommendations that can improve the effects of your prescription and help avoid or reduce the side effects that can sometimes occur with diabetes medicines.

- We'll also check your blood glucose levels with a blood sample taken from your finger, right here in our lab, give you a copy of the results while you're here—and send a copy to your doctor.

- If we should notice anything—either in your blood glucose reading or in what you have to say—that makes us think a change might be indicated, we'll work with you and your doctor to help you achieve the desired goals. We'll also support you in following your diet and exercise programs to help assure that you're getting the best possible results.

- And when it's time for a refill, you can arrange to have that refill waiting when your mini-checkup is finished.

Figure 3. Marketing brochure

Your prescription (along with proper diet and exercise) is intended to help keep your blood glucose under control at all times. And now you can be sure it's doing just that—between your visits to the doctor—at the *Pharmacy Care Center*.

When you enroll in this program, you'll receive regular mini-checkups by a specially trained pharmacist in our *Pharmacy Care Center*. You'll have the results in minutes, and we'll share those results with your doctor.

In no more time than it usually takes for a refill, you'll know whether your blood glucose is under control; get lots of helpful, healthful advice and support from our pharmacists; and be on your way!

And you'll know you're getting the results you should expect—plus the good health and medicine's worth you deserve!

Our *Pharmacy Care Center* Is Especially Important for Patients with Diabetes!

If you follow your doctor's recommendations, eat and exercise properly, and take your medication correctly, your diabetes can be controlled. And the more you know about diabetes and how your medicines work, the more effective that control can be. That's why we recommend regular visits to our *Pharmacy Care Center* between your appointments with the doctor.

Our specially trained pharmacist will work closely with you to:

- give you the facts needed to use your medication correctly—and point out the signs you should look for to avoid possible problems,

- help you organize your medications for easy use,

- provide you with routine checkpoints of your progress towards your diabetes management goals,

- see that you have the information and support you need to make positive changes in your lifestyle, and

- answer any questions you may have about home glucose monitoring—and show you how and when to take blood glucose measurements for the most accurate results.

With our pharmacist's guidance and regular monitoring, your doctor's supervision, and your own active participation, you'll get the best possible results from your medication—for a happier, healthier life!

Figure 3. Marketing brochure (continued)

Physicians/Physician Groups

Having a physician-champion or opinion leader who supports your patient care program is important to your success and essential in developing a health care team approach. Many physicians have not heard of pharmacists providing patient care, so it is important to introduce to physicians the patient care concept and its benefits.

Depending on how your services are paid for, physician referral may be mandatory. However, regardless of whether referral is necessary, it is good policy to keep the physician informed about what you are doing; this leads to two different levels of physician marketing:

- for your information (i.e., this is what I am doing with self-pay patients); and
- send me referrals (i.e., I need referrals because I depend on them to get paid).

Techniques for marketing to physicians will vary with your setting, your relationship with the physicians, and how many physicians are targeted. In some settings, you may have direct access to the primary users of your service, may already have a relationship with these physicians, or may only need to market to a small group. In these cases, the marketing can be done on a personal, one-to-one basis. If you are marketing to a large number of physicians with whom you have had little or no personal contact, a less personal strategy such as a formal marketing letter would be used.

Be careful how you market to physicians. You are likely to encounter the least resistance if you market yourself as an expert assistant and not as a physician replacement. Develop your marketing strategies towards informing physicians of the services you are providing and how they can benefit him or her and the patient. Emphasize that you are working as a part of the health care team to care for patients. The implementation of patient care services should not be contingent on a physician's positive or negative response. Responses will be mixed. Initially, you will need to establish credibility with those who are skeptical.

Identify Physicians to Whom You Wish to Market

Depending on your setting, there are several ways to identify physicians:

- Identify physicians with whom you have an established relationship.
- Identify the physicians of patients who have already been identified.

- Identify the physicians who care for patients with the disease(s) you are specializing in (e.g., family medicine, general medicine, internal medicine, endocrinology, cardiology, pulmonology, allergy, nephrology, etc.).
- Enlist the assistance of the payer of your services to help you identify appropriate physicians.

Contact Identified Physician(s)

If doing one-on-one or small-group marketing, send an introductory letter stating that you will be contacting the physician to make an appointment to discuss the program. A sample letter is included in **Figure 4**. Call the physician's office and set up an appointment with the office manager or reception-ist. Make a point to include as many physicians or staff members (nurses, office manager, etc.) as possible. Organizing a lunch meeting in a group practice is an excellent way to increase your audience size; physicians are accustomed to being provided food when presented with the marketing of a product or service.

At the appointment with the physician(s):

- Introduce yourself and thank him or her for the opportunity to present your program.
- Distribute support materials:
  marketing materials
  business cards
  a menu of services
  a sample patient chart or SOAP note
  a sample physician letter
- Describe the program, its purpose, and goals in verbal and written formats.
- List the benefits of the program. Some example benefits:
  designed to enhance the physician's care
  improves patient adherence to prescribed treatment plan
  helps the patient use his or her medication appropriately
  keeps the physician better informed between visits
- Describe a typical patient interaction.
- Discuss routine physician feedback through the use of summary letters.
- Invite the physician(s) to visit your practice site.
- Make a follow-up telephone call or appointment to receive physician feedback.

Payers

As previously mentioned, the payer may be an insurer, employer, health system, hospital, or

Good Health Pharmacy

411 West Main Street   Stony Brook, VA 23478

December 30, 1997

Jim Belvin, M.D.
Stony Brook Primary Care Physicians, Inc.
789 E. Main Street, Suite #435
Stony Brook, VA 23478

Dear Dr. Belvin,

As I am sure you are aware, several studies show an alarming rate of medication-related hospitalizations, emergency department visits, and physician office visits by patients due to misuse of their medications. To support patients in the proper utilization of their medications, we are offering a new program at Good Health Pharmacy called the Pharmaceutical Care Program. Our goal is to help patients achieve the best possible outcomes from their medication therapy. This is accomplished through drug regimen review, medication regimen compliance and assistance, patient education, and drug therapy monitoring.

I would like to meet with you briefly at your earliest convenience to describe the program in greater detail. I will call your receptionist soon to make an appointment. I look forward to meeting with you.

Sincerely,

Susanne Webster

Susanne Webster, R.Ph.

Figure 4. Sample introductory letter to physician

physician group. Marketing to payers will usually be in the form of proposals and presentations. When marketing to a payer, you will need to present the potential cost benefits of your services and a summary of the literature demonstrating the cost-effectiveness of pharmacist patient care services. You will also need to present, similar to the physician presentation outlined above, the content and benefits of your services. Frequently, both physicians and nonphysicians will be making the decisions about your services. You must present both the clinical and financial objectives of your service. You need to know your audience before making your presentation.

Management

Your marketing efforts to management may include proposals and presentations. Who in management you market your program to will depend on your setting. You should identify the key decision makers. You may need to market beginning with the management level closest to you (i.e., your supervisor or department director) and work your way up to the level within the system responsible for creating and maintaining patient services. For example, in a community pharmacy setting, you may need to discuss a potential program with your immediate supervisor and then a regional manager before proceeding to corporate management. In a hospital-based clinic, you may need to market first to the pharmacy department director, then to the hospital director and financial officer. You may also need to market to the pharmacy and therapeutics committee, administrative council, board of directors, or medical staff committee, depending on who needs to approve a program and any protocols that detail the procedures for the program.

Community Resource Organizations

Depending on your setting and how you get patients into your program, another group you may wish to market to are community resource organizations. Local chapters of health support groups (e.g., American Heart Association and American Diabetes Association) should be informed of your service because you may be referring patients to them and they can refer patients to you. This can be accomplished by a telephone call, an introductory letter, and/or by making an appointment to discuss the program with the head of the organization. An example introductory letter is given in **Figure 5**.

Ongoing Effort

Marketing is an ongoing effort. Although you may initially market to some parties (such as management), you need to think of your services as a business that requires ongoing marketing efforts to all important parties. For example, assume you are in a hospital-based clinic and, based on your initial marketing efforts, management agreed to support your setting up an asthma clinic. You need to periodically let management know the outcomes, both clinical and financial, of the clinic compared with your projections. By reminding them what a good decision this was, you will gain support for expanding your efforts even before you request it.

You also need to assess the outcomes of your marketing efforts. This may include looking at the number of brochures you distributed to patients and the number of patients you discussed services with compared with the number of patients who made an appointment to be seen. You can assess physician referral patterns and identify why you were more successful with some physicians and not others. By assessing the outcomes, you can find ways to improve your marketing.

Case Study

Unihealth is a California health care system that owns hospitals and physician practices and accepts a high percentage of capitated insurance plans. Under the capitated plans, the hospitals and physician practices receive a set amount of money per year for caring for each patient, no matter how many visits or hospitalizations he or she has.

The pharmacy department saw a need for preventing unnecessary hospitalizations among certain patient populations—patients with diabetes, asthma, and cardiovascular disease and patients who were anticoagulated. The pharmacy department chose to begin with an anticoagulation clinic because the system previously had this type of clinic, which was well accepted by the physicians. It was decided to open a clinic at one hospital (Long Beach Community Medical Center) to begin the program.

The pharmacy department identified the following as their primary marketing targets:
- hospital management (chief operating officer, chief financial officer, and medical director)—the payer;

Good Health Pharmacy

411 West Main Street　Stony Brook, VA　23478

December 30, 1997

(name of head of organization)
(name of organization)
(organization address)

Dear (name of head of organization),

As a health care professional, I am aware of the valuable programs and services your organization provides. At Good Health Pharmacy, we are dedicated to the health of the community as well. As part of this dedication, we are offering a new program at our pharmacy, the Pharmaceutical Care Program.

The Pharmaceutical Care Program provides a number of special services for patients who take medications for asthma, diabetes, high blood pressure, or high cholesterol. Our goal is to make sure these patients on long-term therapy get the best results possible from their medication through this special program.

As part of this program, we provide patients with the following:
- private consultations to discuss how their medication is working and any problems or questions they may have;
- regular monitoring of their condition to look for possible side effects and check their progress towards personal health goals; and
- educational material about their condition, the medications they are taking, and how certain activities can help their medications work better.

As part of this new program, we will encounter patients with particular needs that may benefit from community organizations such as (name of organization). If this situation arises, we would like to refer the patients to your organization. As a community organization, you may likewise encounter patients that could benefit from the Pharmaceutical Care Program. We would appreciate any referrals you would like to make to our program as well. If you would like further information concerning our program call 200-0044 or stop by the pharmacy to see what we are doing firsthand.

Sincerely,

SUSANNE WEBSTER

Susanne Webster, R.Ph.

Figure 5. Sample introductory letter to community organization

- the pharmacy and therapeutics (P&T) committee of the hospital (to approve protocols for the clinic);
- house staff physicians; and
- physician groups owned by the system—the customers.

A secondary target was physician groups not owned by the system but who admitted patients to the hospital.

The initial steps in the pharmacy department's marketing plan were to gather data on potential cost savings of the patient care clinics (**Figure 6**, which includes data on anticoagulated patients and patients with other diseases to be targeted in the future) and identify a supportive physician who would be willing to oversee the clinic. Next, they presented the data on the cost savings to hospital management. Once the program was approved, they developed protocols for the clinic and presented the protocols to the overseeing physician and P&T committee for approval. When the protocols where approved, they began marketing to the house staff physicians and system-owned physician groups. The primary method of marketing was letters to each physician detailing the services which would be offered and how to refer patients to the anticoagulation clinic. After marketing to the system-owned physician groups, they conducted similar efforts with the outside physician groups. A sample letter to the physicians is shown in **Figure 7**. Ongoing marketing efforts of the clinic include periodic presentations of the cost-effectiveness data of the clinic to management and occasional reminders to the physician groups. **Table 1** presents some of the preliminary cost savings data from the anticoagulation clinic.

Based on this data, Unihealth calculated projected cost savings of $70,400 per year, or $1717 per patient per year. This cost savings is calculated as follows: If the number of hospital days avoided was 88 days (138 – 50 days) and an estimated cost per hospital day of $400 is used, then the total saved during the initial 6 months of operation was $35,200 (88 days × $400 per day). Extrapolating this to a full year, Unihealth would realize savings of $70,400 ($35,200 × 2). This is equivalent to $1717 per patient per year ($70,400/41 patients).

The pharmacy department is about to open asthma and diabetes clinics. A patient marketing brochure for all three clinics and a physician marketing letter are shown in **Figures 8** and **9**.

Summary

No matter who your target groups are or which methods you choose, the most important thing to do is begin marketing efforts immediately. Once underway, evaluate the effectiveness of your marketing by soliciting comments and suggestions from patients and other health care providers. Be flexible and persistent. Every practice setting will be different and you alone know what works best in your setting.

Reference

1. Hepler CD, Strand LM. Opportunities and responsibilities in pharmaceutical care. *Am J Pharm Educ* 1989;53:7S–15S.

Table 1. Health Management Center Cost Savings Study Data

	6 Months Before	6 Months During	% Decrease
Number of Patients	41	41	0
Total Hospital Admissions	21	11	47.6
Total Hospital Days	138	50	63.8
Hospital Days/Patient	3.37	1.22	63.8
Total Emergency Room Visits	4	4	0

ANTICIPATED SAVINGS AND COST ANALYSIS

LABORATORY COST PROJECTIONS	Estimated % per Disease	Estimated % per Disease	Annual Variable Cost/
	Year 1	Year 2	Disease
Asthma	5%	5%	$ 0.00
Hypertension	0%	3%	$ 0.00
Diabetes Mellitus	5%	10%	$18.00
Hyperlipidemia	0%	7%	$30.98
Hypertension + Diabetes	2%	5%	$21.15
Hypertension + Hyperlipidemia	0%	4%	$30.98
Hyperlipidemia + Diabetes	3%	6%	$52.03
Hypertens. + Hyperlipid. + Diab.	0%	2%	$52.03
Fragmin	10%	10%	$72.00
Anticoagulation	75%	48%	$72.00
	100%	100%	

Fixed Cost Projections

Pharmacists labor cost fixed at:
40 hours per week × 52 weeks @ $48.25 per hour
per Pharm.D. $100,360

Administrative Assistant $25,000

Annual Patient Flow and Variable Cost

	Number of Patients/Year	Annual Variable Cost
Lab costs for comprehensive patients		
Year 1	150	$ 9,613
Year 2	300	$15,656

Financial Assumptions

Investment financed (start-up costs)	$18,829
Interest rate	7%
Term (yr)	2
Annual interest and amortization	$10,414
Overhead (% of total program cost)	5%

Projected Savings Analysis

	Year 1	Year 2	Total
Projected Savings			
Savings from Anticoag patients $950 per patient per year	$106,875	$136,800	$243,675
Savings from Fragmin patients, $3200 per patient per year	$ 48,000	$ 96,000	$144,000
Savings from patients with other conditions, $650 pppy	$ 14,625	$ 81,900	$ 96,525
TOTAL	$169,500	$314,700	$484,200

Figure 6. Anticipated savings and cost analysis

Costs

Labor costs	$125,360	$125,360	$250,720
Laboratory cost	$ 9,613	$ 15,656	$ 25,269
Maintenance fee for software	$ 2,640	$ 2,640	$ 5,280
TOTAL	$137,613	$143,656	$281,269

Operating Savings (Loss) $31,887 $171,044 $202,931

Overhead	$ 0	$ 0	$ 0
Interest and Amortization	$ 10,414	$ 10,414	$ 20,828

Savings After Interest and Amortization $21,473 $160,630 $182,103

Number of patients in program year 1	150
Number of patients in program year 2	300
Dollar savings per anticoag patient	950
Dollar savings per Fragmin patient	3200
Dollar savings per patient, other disease states	650
Software maintenance fee per year	2640
Pharmacist cost per hour	48.25
Number of Pharm.D. hours per week	40

Figure 6. Anticipated savings and cost analysis (continued)

Long Beach Community Medical Center

November 5, 1997

Dear Doctor,

We are pleased to announce the reopening of the Coumadin/Anticoagulation Clinic at Long Beach Community Medical Center. We are located in the Education Pavilion at 4290 E. Pacific Coast Highway on the turning circle. We are here to assist you with your patients' anticoagulation needs.

The Coumadin Clinic offers "Point of Care Testing" with Protimes being performed by finger stick. Patients receive their INR results before they leave the clinic. Our Protime Point of Care System is certified.

The clinical pharmacist reviews the results with the patient, and dosage changes, if needed, are discussed to bring the patient's INR to within the range you have chosen. The patient receives a typed information sheet of his or her dosing schedule and the date he or she is to return for the next INR test. In addition, patients are tracked using Dupont's software program, CoumaCare. We will be providing you with copies of progress notes within 24 hours to keep you well informed on how your patient is doing. So far, we have received overwhelmingly positive feedback from patients and referring physicians.

We are also pleased to announce that we will be treating Outpatients with Low Molecular Weight Heparin (Fragmin®) for Acute Deep Venous Thrombosis. We will be working in conjunction with the patient's primary care physician, the hospital's emergency room physician, and Clinishare.

Clinic Hours: Monday–Friday: 0800–1800
                  Weekends, Holidays, and after hours: On Call

On behalf of our staff, we look forward to working with you and your patients to improve their satisfaction and compliance by having them participate in their own health management process.

To refer a patient, please call us at 200-0044 or fax referral form to 200-0045.

We are enclosing several blank referral forms. Please call us for additional forms or photocopy them as you find convenient.

Sincerely,

Terry Rubin

Terry Rubin, Pharm.D.
Pharmacist Clinic Manager

Marvin Appel

Marvin Appel, M.D., F.A.C.C.
Physician Clinic Administrator

Figure 7. Unihealth physician marketing letter, example 1

The Health Management Center

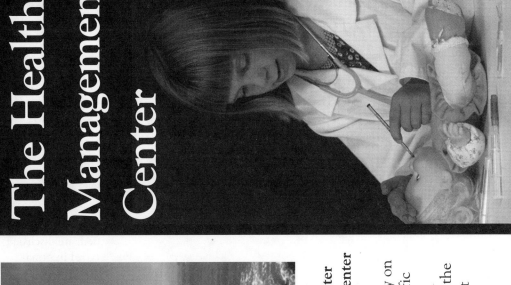

LONG BEACH COMMUNITY MEDICAL CENTER

The Health Management Center of Long Beach Community Center is located at:

4290 E. Pacific Coast Highway on the Lakewood Boulevard–Pacific Coast Highway Traffic Circle.

For more information, contact the **Health Management Center** at

(562) 498-4526

or visit our website at **www.lbommunity.com.**

HOW CAN THE HEALTH MANAGEMENT CENTER HELP ME?

The Health Management Center will enhance the good care you receive from your physician. Results of your laboratory tests will be reviewed with you during each visit. We have a dietitian and a diabetic nurse educator available to meet with you, if needed. Every time you visit the Health Management Center, you will receive a medication plan and dosing schedule. This will provide you with the instruction and education you need to optimize your medicine and reduce the risks of side effects.

WHAT CLINICS ARE CURRENTLY AVAILABLE?

The Health Management Center currently offers three clinics:

- anticoagulation
- asthma
- diabetes

The following clinics are scheduled to open in the near future:

- congestive heart failure
- hyperlipidemia

Figure 8. Unihealth patient marketing brochure

THE HEALTH MANAGEMENT CENTER OF LONG BEACH COMMUNITY MEDICAL CENTER

OFFERS A *NEW* APPROACH FOR PATIENTS

WHO REQUIRE PRECISE MONITORING OF THEIR MEDICATION

Patients who require continued monitoring of anticoagulation, asthma, or diabetes medication now have the Health Management Center available to them. The center provides education, monitoring of medications, and self-management training in an outpatient setting.

The Health Management Center uses state-of-the-art laboratory analyzers that require only one drop of blood taken from a finger. Patients receive their test results within minutes!

Our goal at the Health Management Center is to provide our patients with the highest quality care while working closely with their physician to improve their quality of life.

WHAT IS THE PURPOSE OF THE HEALTH MANAGEMENT CENTER?

The purpose of the Health Management Center is to allow our patients to remain free of acute and chronic symptoms and/or complications of their disease. We do this by involving them in all aspects of their health management.

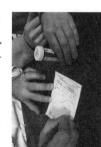

WHAT SETS THE HEALTH MANAGEMENT CENTER APART FROM OTHERS?

We are the only outpatient Health Management Center in Long Beach. The Long Beach Community Medical Center's Health Management Center is staffed by a doctor of pharmacy (Pharm. D.) and a doctor of medicine (M.D.) Patients are seen in a friendly and caring atmosphere. We believe that our patients are the most important members of our health care team. Our primary goal is to keep our patients healthy so they can enjoy life without having any health-related complications.

We will also be working closely with local community pharmacies to ensure quality follow-up care when prescriptions are filled.

The Health Management Center's Administrative Director is Marvin Appel, M.D. Dr. Appel is a nationally renowned expert in cardiology and internal medicine. The center is managed by Terry Rubin, Pharm. D. Dr. Rubin has over 20 years' experience as a manager/clinical specialist in the Long Beach area.

WHAT IS THE COST OF TREATMENT?

There is *no* cost to you or your physician for your treatment. Treatment at the Health Management Center is covered by most insurance plans.

WHAT CAN YOU EXPECT?

Your first visit to the Health Management Center will take approximately one hour. You will meet with a doctor of pharmacy (Pharm. D.) who will take a thorough medication and medical history. Educational materials will be reviewed, including instruction on use of home glucometers and peak flow meters.

Baseline measurements and laboratory results will also be obtained. You will receive a medication plan explained verbally during your visit and a written plan when you leave. The written plan will cover:

- each medication's purpose,
- the proper administration technique for each medication,
- the proper dose to take and when to take it, and
- health goals and reminders.

Follow-up visits to the Health Management Center will take about 15–20 minutes.

HOW DO I MAKE AN APPOINTMENT?

You may be referred to the Health Management Center by your primary care physician or specialist. They can arrange for a referral appointment.

For more information, contact us directly at (562) 498-4526.

Figure 8. Unihealth patient marketing brochure (continued)

Long Beach Community Medical Center

December 30, 1997

Dear Doctor:

We are pleased to announce the expansion of the Health Management Center (HMC) at Long Beach Community Medical Center. In addition to our Anticoagulation program, we have expanded our services to include programs to monitor asthma and diabetes patients.

The goal of the **Asthma Program** is to keep patients free of acute and chronic symptoms through education and motivation. The goal of the **Diabetes Program** is to educate and motivate patients to prevent long-term complications while maintaining blood glucose and hemoglobin A_{1c} levels as close to your goals as possible. These programs meet national treatment guidelines.

We will continue to offer point-of-care testing. We will take finger stick samples of blood for Protimes, glucose levels, and hemoglobin A_{1c}.

The Health Management Center clinical pharmacist will monitor medications and provide self-management training to prevent emergency room visits, hospitalizations, and adverse drug reactions. In addition, we will be working closely with community pharmacies to ensure follow-up care while monitoring prescriptions and refills.

There will be no charge to you or your patient for this service. We will also keep you well informed about how your patients are doing by faxing copies of progress notes to your office after each patient visit.

To refer a patient, please call us at (562) 498-4526 or fax a completed copy of the enclosed referral form to (562) 498-4479.

We believe that these programs will improve patient satisfaction and compliance by increasing patient participation in the health management process. We look forward to assisting you with the care of your diabetes and asthma patients.

Very truly yours,

Terry Rubin

Terry Rubin, Pharm.D.
Pharmacist Clinic Manager

Marvin Appel

Marvin Appel, M.D.
Physician Clinic Administrator

Figure 9. Unihealth physician marketing letter, example 2

Self-Study Questions

Objective

Identify target audiences when marketing your services.

1. Define potential users and payers for your services and describe the reason for targeting marketing efforts to both groups.

2. Which of following best describes why it is important to direct marketing to physicians rather than patients in HMO, clinic, and doctor's office settings.
    A. It demonstrates your dedication to patient care.
    B. The physician must refer patients to your services.
    C. It improves the collaborative relationship between the pharmacist and the physician.
    D. Patients are not influenced by marketing, therefore it is best to target the physician.

3. Describe why it is necessary to market your services to many groups in a community or retail setting.

Objective

Describe elements of an effective marketing plan.

4. Describe how marketing efforts may change over time.

5. Marketing to patients, it is most important to stress:
    A. that your services are less expensive than the physician's services.
    B. the hours that your services are available.
    C. how your services can benefit the patient's disease management.
    D. the cost of your services.

6. Explain why providing free introductory services is a good incentive to encourage patient participation.

7. Which of the following best describes the use of a program logo and name.
    A. A program logo and name are not necessary elements of a marketing plan.
    B. A program logo and name make marketing brochures and letters more attractive.
    C. An attractive program logo provides a competitive edge against others who provide similar services.
    D. A program logo and name allows patients to distinguish your services from those provided by others.

8. All of the following are effective marketing methods when targeting physicians *except*:
    A. letters.
    B. face-to-face meetings.
    C. telephone calls.
    D. newspaper ads.

9. Describe how the tools and approaches used in marketing to payers and management are similar.

Self-Study Answers

1. Users of your services include patients, physicians, and the management of health care systems and businesses. It is important to market to this group because these individuals must participate for you to get paid. Payers for your services include those who are at risk for the cost of drug-related morbidity. These include patients, employers, third-party payers, physician groups, health care systems, and the government. This group is an important target audience because they should be willing to pay to avoid these consequences.

2. B

3. In the community or retail setting, it is important to market to more groups because the potential payers for your services are any party at risk for health care costs, including patients, employers, third-party payers, physician groups, health care systems, and the government.

4. Marketing efforts for a new service may initially target management, patients, and physicians.

After you have proven the value of your services to management, you may only need to reinforce this with periodic marketing efforts. Marketing to patients and physicians is usually a continual process.

5. C

6. Free introductory services, such as screenings, allow the patient to experience the potential benefits of your services. They also give you the opportunity to describe the importance and scope of your services and demonstrate your dedication to patient care.

7. D

8. D

9. Effective marketing tools to payers and management include proposals and presentations. Marketing efforts to both groups should demonstrate the potential benefits of your services, including cost savings and clinical benefits.

Creating and Maintaining a Patient Tracking System

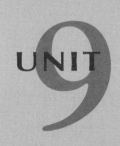

Tracking patient activity services is a management and patient care tool. As a management tool, a patient tracking system allows monitoring of pharmacist productivity and selection of patients for quality assurance monitoring. If more than one pharmacist is seeing patients, you can create pharmacist "report cards" to compare patient loads and time utilization. Using the tracking system, you can select patients for quality assurance monitoring by such categories as pharmacist, disease, or last visit. The records of the identified patients can then be reviewed according to the standards of your quality assurance monitoring program. A tracking system allows you to select patients or physicians for assessing acceptance of your services. As a patient care tool, a patient tracking system helps to promote proactive care by allowing you to identify patients requiring follow-up. Also, it allows identification of a pharmacist's effort at keeping the physician informed of the patient's condition.

Unit Objectives

After you successfully complete this unit, you will be able to:
- explain methods of tracking patients in an ambulatory pharmacy service,
- list elements commonly found in a patient tracking system, and
- describe uses of a patient tracking system.

Unit Organization

This unit begins with a discussion of tools available to track patient care services. Information that should be recorded in the chosen system is then specified. Next, the process of patient tracking and possible applications of the data are described. The unit concludes with a presentation of methods to update the system.

Tools for Tracking Patients

Patient tracking can be accomplished manually or electronically. Manual patient tracking is performed using a patient tracking form. An example is included in **Figure 1**. A software spreadsheet program such as Microsoft Excel, Lotus 1-2-3, or Quattro Pro or database programs such as Microsoft

Access can be used to track patients electronically. Although electronic tracking requires computer software and the knowledge to use it, it is less cumbersome to use and information is easier to retrieve than from a manual system, especially if you have a large number of patients.

Items to Track

Some items you should consider tracking include:
- patient name;
- enrollment or initial visit date;
- date of most recent visit;
- total number of interventions to date;
- referral source;
- reason for referral;
- physician name;
- total number of pharmacist communications with physician;
- type of communications (telephone, letter, or in person);
- name of pharmacist (if more than one person is seeing patients);
- patient status (active or closed); and
- disease states.

Other items can be added to this list, depending on your specific needs. For example, as will be discussed in unit 11, Providing Quality Care, you may wish to use your patient tracking system to also track patient outcomes. For example, you might track hemoglobin A_{1c} and fasting glucose values for diabetic patients and blood pressure for hypertension patients.

Process

Information in the patient tracking system should be updated after each patient interaction and after communicating with a patient's health care providers. Review the patient tracking list at least once a week so you can contact patients who need follow-up.

To effectively follow up on patients, the following steps need to be taken. At the end of each workday, for patients seen that day, update:
- date patient last seen,
- patient status, and
- physician communication.

Each week, you should:
- Review the "date patient last seen" column to identify patients who have not been seen in the maximum period of time between

Patient Tracking Form

Patient Name	ID#	Status	Enroll Date	Last Visit	Inter-ven-tions	Pharmacist	Physician	Physician Contacts	Type of Contact	Disease State(s)	Reason for Referral
Bennett, Emma	2347	A	4/12/98	3/18/99	3	Clark	Taylor	5	L = 3 C=2	Asthma	Nonadher-ence
Smith, Samuel	3487	A	5/28/98	1/18/99	4	Clark	Stevens	3	L = 3	Diabetes	Uncontrolled
Jones, Herbert	8567	A	1/12/99	1/12/99	0	Henry	Stevens	0		HTN Diabetes	Uncontrolled
Collins, Josephine	1897	A	2/18/99	3/18/99	1	Henry	Banks	1	C = 1	Asthma	Nonadher-ence
TOTALS 4					8			9	L = 6 C = 3		

Status: A = active; C = closed
Type of communication: L = letter; C = telephone call; P = in person

Figure 1. Example Patient Tracking Form—March 1999

visits you set. This interval will depend on your setting. For example, in an anticoagulation clinic you may decide that patients must be seen at least every 6 weeks.

- Retrieve records of identified patients and determine the reason for their having not been seen. If a patient has no scheduled follow-up appointment, call to reschedule and complete documentation of the rescheduled appointment.

Examine **Figure 1** again. Assume this report is for the end of March. Based on an every-6-week visit interval, which patients need to have their records reviewed? You should review the charts of Mr. Smith and Mr. Jones to determine why they have not been seen since January. The records may reveal a reason, such as that the patient had an interim physician visit and did not need to be seen or that the patient was going to be out of town for an extended period and has a follow-up appointment scheduled in April. Another reason may be that the pharmacist determined the patient was stable and did not need to be seen every 6 weeks. If either patient does not have a follow-up appointment, one needs to be scheduled.

An alternative method of preventing patients from being lost to follow-up is to add a column for next appointment date to your tracking form. You can examine this column for patients without appointments or who have missed an appointment as indicated by a date that has passed.

Updating the Patient Tracking System

There are numerous ways to keep the information up to date in your patient tracking system. If using a computerized format, you can print a hard copy of the patient tracking form for daily updates or enter the updates directly into the computer program. For example, when using a hard copy form, update information manually at the end of each day. When new patients are seen, add their names and patient information in blank spaces at the end of the hard copy of the patient tracking form. Use the hard copy to update the electronic patient tracking system on a monthly or weekly basis.

Summary

Tracking patients is important for maintaining information on the patients you provide care for and preventing patients from being lost to follow-up. A patient tracking system can be as simple as a paper form for a small number of patients to a computerized database for larger patient populations.

Self-Study Questions

Objective

Explain methods of tracking patients in an ambulatory pharmacy service.

1. Describe available tools to track patient information and give an example of each.

Objective

List elements commonly found in a patient tracking system.

2. Which of the following is an example of demographic or administrative data that may be recorded in the patient tracking system?
   A. laboratory results
   B. current medication regimen
   C. disease states
   D. physician name

3. Which of the following is not an outcomes measure that may be recorded in the patient tracking system?
   A. number of interventions
   B. blood pressure
   C. hemoglobin A_{1c}
   D. total cholesterol

Objective

Describe uses of a patient tracking system.

4. Explain possible uses of a patient tracking system.

Self-Study Answers

1. Patient information may be tracked through the use of manual and electronic tools. Manual tracking uses a paper form with columns for each piece of information. Electronic tools, including programs such as Microsoft Excel, Lotus 1-2-3, or Quattro Pro, use spreadsheets to track and retrieve information.

2. D

3. A

4. The main use of a patient tracking system is to confirm that patients receive follow-up treatment. It identifies patients who have not been seen during the maximum time period set by your service so they can be contacted for an appointment. A patient tracking system can also be used to track pharmacist productivity and for quality assurance monitoring.

Legal Issues

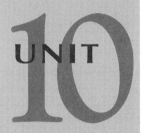

When providing patient care services, the pharmacist assumes greater responsibility for patient outcomes. With greater responsibility comes accountability and the potential for liability. This possibility should not create fear, nor deter you from practicing pharmaceutical care. The true value of your contributions will not be recognized until you are willing to take responsibility for your actions.

Some simple measures should be taken to help decrease potential liability. These measures include:

- patient release statements,
- liability insurance,
- documentation,
- maintaining patient confidentiality, and
- awareness of medical-legal concepts.

Unit Objectives

After you successfully complete this unit, you will be able to:

- describe measures to reduce the potential for liability when providing patient care services,
- state the medical-legal concepts that apply when providing care in an ambulatory patient care service, and
- explain the need to maintain patient confidentiality.

Unit Organization

This unit begins with a discussion of methods to decrease liability when providing ambulatory patient care, including patient consent forms, liability insurance, and proper documentation. Next, medical-legal concepts that apply to the pharmacist-patient relationship are explained. Finally, the importance of patient confidentiality and tips for maintaining it are described.

Patient Release Statements

One of the most effective ways to reduce your liability is to routinely use a consent form to explain the responsibilities of the pharmacist and your services. This form should also contain a clause that releases you from liability associated with drawing blood and releasing patient information to the patient's other health care providers and insurance company. Because of patient confidentiality of information, you need the patient's permission before releasing or discussing their information with other parties.

Figure 1 shows a sample consent form. A blank form for your use can be found in **Appendix 1**. Review the consent form with the patient and make sure he or she understands it fully. Patients should sign a consent form before any information is obtained from them. File the signed form in the patient's record.

Depending on your setting, patients may have already signed a consent form or release of information form. Release of information forms are commonly used in clinics, physician's offices, and HMOs. If your site uses its own form, keep the original signed consent in the patient's record.

Liability Insurance

You should check your personal or employer-provided professional liability insurance plan to make sure you have adequate coverage for your type of practice. Usually, if your activities fit within the current definition of pharmacy practice within your state, the insurer would cover the claim. Pharmacy practice acts and regulations do vary from state to state. You can check with your state board of pharmacy regarding its regulations about your services. You can submit a detailed written description of your activities to the professional liability insurance company and request a written response as to whether these activities would be covered.[1] Maintain copies of all correspondence with the insurance company for future reference.

Consider purchasing personal professional liability insurance, regardless of whether your employer covers you.[2] Most professional pharmacy organizations offer programs for purchasing such insurance as a member benefit.

Documentation

Appropriate documentation is one of the best ways to reduce the risk of liability. Remember: "If it wasn't documented, it wasn't done." Activities that should routinely be documented were discussed in unit 6. This unit discusses documenting drug-related problems, pharmacist-physician disagreements, and terminating pharmacist-patient relationships.

PATIENT RELEASE STATEMENT

I understand that my Good Health Pharmacy pharmacist will be working to help me improve and maintain my health through a better understanding of my health problems and helping me make the most effective use of my medications. As part of this process, Good Health Pharmacy will provide health-related information about me and the services I have received to my physicians to keep them informed of my progress and will provide information necessary for billing to my insurance company.

I hereby authorize Good Health Pharmacy to release to my physician and insurance company, _Blue Cross/Blue Shield_, all information and records related to the care I receive.

I understand that a portion of Good Health Pharmacy's service includes my giving a series of blood samples for the purpose of monitoring. There may be some discomfort, bruising, bleeding, or swelling at the puncture site and surrounding tissue, and it may become infected. If I see signs of infection (redness, swelling, warmth, pain, or pus), I will seek medical care from my physician.

I hereby release Good Health Pharmacy, their affiliates, directors, officers, employees, successors, and assigns from any and all liability arising from or in any way connected with this release of such information and with this blood drawing. I understand that I should not participate in these tests if I suffer from any bleeding disorder or similar condition.

Date: _1/13/98_

Printed name: _Sarah Mistler_

Signature: _Sarah Mistler_

Figure 1. Sample consent form

Documenting Pharmacotherapeutic and Related Health Care Problems

When you begin providing more direct patient care, you will most likely discover more pharmacotherapeutic and related health care problems than ever before. It is essential to document the problem and the action taken to correct the situation. When documenting a pharmacotherapeutic and related health care problem, avoid using words that imply blame or substandard care on the part of any health care professional, health care institution, or manufacturer. See **Table 1** for a list of words to avoid. Document only facts and not a patient's interpretation of care. Your description of a problem should be as accurate, concise, and objective as possible. Limit your description to what happened and avoid explaining, rationalizing, or arguing your case in the patient's record.

Here is an example of documentation (a SOAP [Subjective, Objective, Assessment, Plan] note) that includes a potential problem:

S: Patient seen in pharmacy care center today for blood pressure check after recent diltiazem dose increase. Patient complains of dizziness on standing and has had one fall. Patient complained of dizziness when she stood for standing blood pressure measurement.

O: BP = 130/88, sitting pulse = 65   BP = 110/68, standing pulse = 72

A: Orthostatic hypotension leading to fall is due to inappropriate dose of diltiazem prescribed by Dr. Smith.

P: Told patient her dose was excessive. Will call Dr. Smith.

The SOAP note above states that Dr. Smith is at fault for this patient's fall. Although the patient's orthostatic hypotension is likely a result of an excessive dose, this effect of the dose is not a fact.

Here is an improved version:

S: Patient seen in pharmacy care center today for blood pressure check after recent diltiazem dose increase. Patient complains of dizziness on standing and has had one fall. Patient complained of dizziness when she stood for standing blood pressure measurement.

O: BP = 130/88, sitting pulse = 65   BP = 110/68, standing pulse = 72

A: Orthostatic hypotension

P: Will discuss with Dr. Smith. Patient was told her blood pressure was dropping on standing and was educated about strategies to minimize problems with blood pressure changes when changing positions.

The differences in the two SOAP notes may seem subtle, but the second example does not speculate on the cause of the lowered blood pressure, it only states the facts as known. Put yourself in the position of an unbiased outsider when proofread-

Table 1. Words to Avoid in Medical Records

Words That Imply Substandard Care or Performance

aberrant	problem
bad	sloppy
defective	substandard
faulty	undesirable
inadequate	unsatisfactory
inappropriate	wrong
incorrect	
insufficient	
poor	

Words That Imply Blame

accidental	misadventure
blame	mistake
careless	mix-up
confused	negligent
erroneous	regret
error	regretful
fault	sorry
foolish	terrible
inadvertent	unfortunate

Source: reprinted from *Ambulatory Care Clinical Skills Program: Core Module.* Bethesda, MD: American Society of Health-System Pharmacists; 1998. p. 27.

ing each of your notes, to detect any potentially problematic phrases and to assess the general tone of the note. Remember that patient records are legal documents and can be used in lawsuits against you or other health care providers.

Pharmacist-Physician Disagreement

A pharmacist-physician disagreement occurs when a physician insists on prescribing a regimen or medication with which the pharmacist does not agree. In such a situation, you should notify the physician of potential problems and document this communication. In most instances, the pharmacist can then defer to the physician's expertise and not run into legal problems. However, if the potential exists for great harm or death to the patient, you are responsible for warning the physician of the gravity of the situation. In this case, your actions should be guided by the welfare of the patient. Again, documentation is imperative.

Awareness of Medical-Legal Concepts

In providing care directly to the patient, you establish a professional relationship with the patient and should be aware of certain medical-legal concepts, such as duty to care, terminating the relationship, abandonment, and harmful neglect.

Duty to Care

When you begin providing services to a patient, you establish a pharmacist-patient relationship that gives rise to the duty to care. This contractual agreement is between you and the patient, rather than between the patient and the physician, as is often the view of traditional pharmacy practice. Negligence occurs when you are under a duty to a patient to use due care, you breach that duty, and the breach directly results in the patient suffering damages.

Terminating the Relationship

If the pharmacist-patient relationship has been formed and is to be terminated, for whatever reason, you must give the patient sufficient notice so he or she may obtain other professional care. As a pharmacist, your power in terminating the relationship is relatively limited. For example, the patient's failure to cooperate with treatment may be sufficient cause for you to terminate the professional relationship; however, you must carefully document refusal

of treatment before terminating the relationship. Offer to help the patient make alternative care arrangements, such as referring him or her back to the physician if necessary.

The patient, on the other hand, has more power in terminating the relationship and may do so at any time. From the moment the pharmacist is dismissed or discharged, he or she is relieved of all future professional responsibility to the patient.

Abandonment

Abandonment is considered to have occurred if the following are proved:

- the existence of a pharmacist-patient relationship,
- the pharmacist has unilaterally severed the relationship without reasonable notice and without providing an adequate substitute,
- the patient requires (or did require) continuing pharmaceutical attention,
- the patient suffered damages, and
- proximate cause (damages and the severed relationship are closely related in time).

In essence, you must continue to provide services to a patient who needs your services and with whom you have established a relationship. You may terminate the relationship if you give the patient sufficient notice so he or she may find alternative care. Document that you gave the patient sufficient notice and a referral to alternative care.

Harmful Neglect

If something happens to a patient between visits, the pharmacist may come under scrutiny for harmful neglect. Only if there is a factual link between a pharmacist's actions and a patient's injury and it is deemed that the pharmacist could have foreseen the potential harm would harmful neglect be considered. Harmful neglect encompasses both actions that the pharmacist performs and those that he or she fails to perform. For example, if a pharmacist increases a patient's warfarin dose after obtaining a falsely low international normalized ratio (INR) value without first evaluating the patient's clinical presentation, this could be considered harmful neglect if this action results in patient injury. A pharmacist might be suspected of harmful neglect because of an omitted action, for example, if he or she fails to counsel a patient with hypertension about disease-drug interactions that can occur with nonprescription decongestants and the patient suffers a severe adverse effect after using one of these products.

Documentation of encounters with patients and follow-up recommendations are important. On the other hand, patients have the responsibility of following reasonable treatment plans.

Communicating with Patients About Drug-Related Problems

Avoid implying blame, negligence, or substandard care by yourself or another health care professional when talking with patients. This can be particularly important when a drug-related problem has harmed the patient, but no professional negligence occurred. Reasonable errors of professional judgment do occur but are not the same as negligence. Negligence is failure to exercise the degree of care considered reasonable under the circumstances, resulting in an unintended injury.

When explaining drug-related problems to patients, observe the following to avoid implying blame, negligence, or substandard care:

- Be certain the patient understands that a problem has occurred.
- Never alter the facts to minimize the problem.
- Explain the cause of the problem in the most accurate way.
- Beware of speculating on the cause of the problem.
- Avoid using problem words, such as those found in **Table 1** (e.g., "I regret that this happened").
- Avoid discussing drug-related problems as unavoidable.
- Avoid exaggerated and inaccurate characterizations of the problem (e.g., saying "That reaction is very, very rare" when the reaction is not rare).
- Show concern for the patient with drug-related problems.

Patient Confidentiality

Patients have entrusted you with the privilege of, and authority for, their care. Part of this process is your responsibility to maintain strict patient confidentiality at all times. Patient information is confidential and protected by law. You must be cognizant of all verbal, written, and stored patient information to avoid betrayal of this confidence.

What Information Is Confidential?

The three-zone confidentiality model in **Figure 2** illustrates the sensitivity levels of patient information. Based on this model, some information is designated as not necessarily confidential, but some patients may prefer that all their information remain confidential.

Avoid Patient-Specific Conversations

Avoid patient-specific conversations in public places and anywhere within hearing range of non–health care team members. Be aware of where you conduct patient-specific telephone conversations with patients and health care providers. These interactions must be conducted in private areas. Do not discuss patients with colleagues in the dispensing area or other public areas. You may be overheard, and you will not portray a professional image. A good rule of thumb is to put yourself in the patient's place.

Maintain Patient Confidentiality

The patient's record documents many aspects of that person's health status; therefore, precautions must be taken to keep this information confidential. Records must not be left in public view, and users of electronic medical records should make sure to completely exit the electronic record before leaving the patient care area. Passwords should be maintained in strict confidence. If used, hard-copy records should be filed and maintained in a restricted area.

State laws are not consistent on how long records need to be maintained. If computerized records are ever destroyed, you must ensure that all data are fully destroyed (including any backup copies of records) and that confidentiality of the records is preserved. Disposal of electronic medical records is an issue when having an outside person destroy them or when disposing of the remains of records (e.g., shredded documents).

Maintaining Patient Records

Here are some suggestions for handling patient records:

- Restrict access to the records and computer system.
- Warn, educate, and train users (consider having a policy on confidentiality that is distributed yearly).
- If using computerized medical records, perform frequent data backups.
- When destroying records, destroy data completely (including backups).
- Protect against computer viruses (do not allow unknown disks and software to be

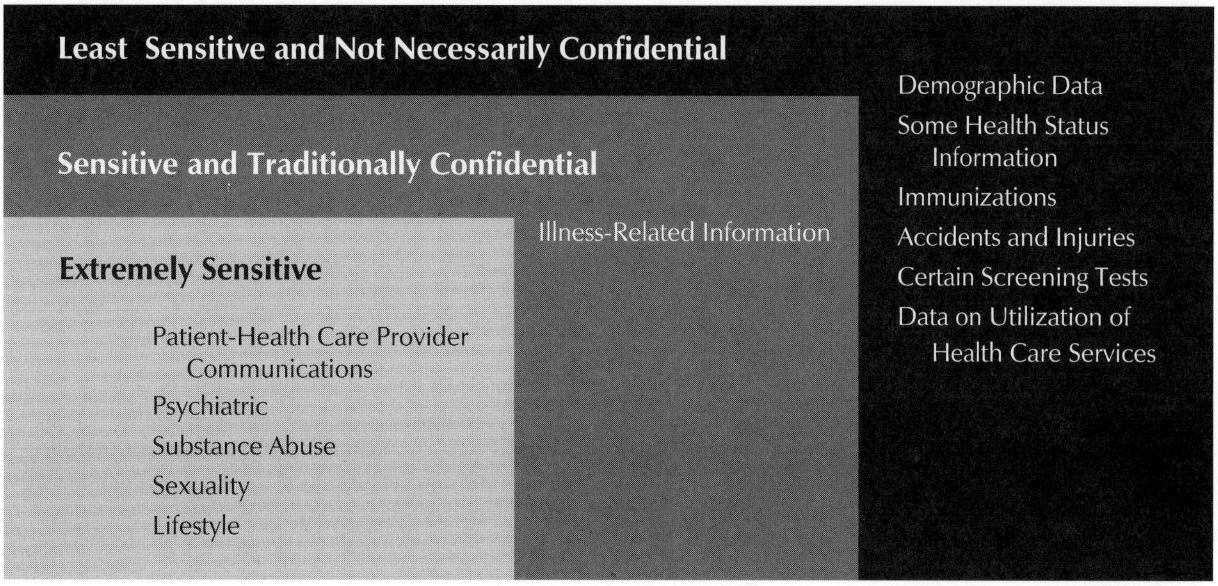

Figure 2. Three-zone confidentiality model

Source: Dick RS, Steen EB, editors. *The Computer-Based Medical Record: An Essential Technology for Health Care*. Washington, DC: National Academy Press; 1991. p.84.

installed or used; check for viruses frequently).

• Use common sense.

Awareness of the issue of confidentiality and common sense are needed to avoid unauthorized disclosure of confidential information. Any betrayal of patient confidentiality is a breach of the patient's right to privacy and can result in destruction of the pharmacist-patient relationship, jeopardy of patient care, and legal action.

Summary

The increasing responsibility of pharmacists for patient outcomes brings with it increased accountability. Accountability is important to becoming a

valued member of a patient's health care team. The increased risk of liability can be greatly reduced by simple measures, such as appropriate documentation of activities, routine use of patient release statements, maintenance of patient confidentiality, and awareness of your responsibilities once a relationship is established with a patient. In addition, you should be certain that you have adequate insurance coverage for your pharmaceutical care services.

References

1. Fink JL. Does expanded role mean greater expectations? *Am Druggist* 1997; June: 59–65.
2. Williams KG. Liability for expanded responsibilities. *Am J Health Syst Pharm* 1997;54:1152, 1157.

Self-Study Questions

Objective
Describe measures to reduce the potential for liability when providing patient care services.

1. All of the following are effective ways to reduce your liability risk *except:*
   A. patient consent forms.
   B. adequate liability insurance.
   C. staff legal counsel.
   D. documentation.

2. Which of the following best describes the role of the patient consent form?
   A. It allows you to access patient medical records.
   B. It prevents the patient from filing legal claims against you, regardless of the circumstance.
   C. It can be sent to the patient's insurance provider to justify reimbursement for service.
   D. It explains your responsibilities, allows you to access patient records, and decreases your liability.

3. Explain how the tone and terminology used in documentation can be used to decrease liability.

4. Describe how to document disagreements that occur between the pharmacist and the physician providing care.

Objective
State the medical-legal concepts that apply when providing care in an ambulatory patient care service.

5. Describe what is meant by the term *duty to care.*

6. The power to terminate the pharmacist-patient relationship belongs primarily to:
   A. the pharmacist.
   B. the patient's insurance provider.
   C. the patient's legal counsel.
   D. the patient.

7. Which of the following best describes the termination of a pharmacist-patient relationship when the patient fails to cooperate?
   A. You may terminate the relationship without notice because it was the patient's choice to refuse your services.
   B. You need only document the patient's refusal of services.
   C. You should document the patient's refusal of care and refer the patient to alternative services.
   D. You have no right to terminate the pharmacist-patient relationship, under any circumstance.

Objective
Explain the need to maintain patient confidentiality.

8. Which of the following information is considered least sensitive and therefore not necessarily confidential?
   A. immunization status
   B. illness-related information
   C. lifestyle information
   D. history of illegal substance use

9. Describe how patient confidentiality can be maintained when using electronic patient records.

Self-Study Answers

1. C

2. D

3. Patient records are legal documents; your documentation should include only the known facts, not subjective statements or conjecture. Avoid using words that imply blame or a substandard level of care.

4. Should you disagree with a physician's recommendation, explain the potential problems and the gravity of the situation, if necessary. All communication should be documented.

5. The duty to care is a contractual agreement to provide care that exists between the patient and the pharmacist. The pharmacist may be guilty of negligence if this duty is breached and it results in the patient suffering harm.

6. D

7. C

8. A

9. Employees accessing electronic patient medical records should confirm that they have completely exited the medical record before leaving the patient care area. Passwords should also be confidential. When deleting electronic medical records, ensure the data is completely destroyed and that the party completing this destruction maintains the confidentiality of the information.

Providing Quality Care

UNIT

11

When providing patient care services, you want to ensure that you are providing quality care that is achieving the desired outcomes. Providing quality care to patients is important for many reasons, including professional satisfaction, accreditation and reimbursement purposes, identification of areas for staff education, and justification for continuing and expanding services.

The goal of quality improvement and outcomes monitoring is to understand and continuously improve all the processes in delivery of patient care. To accomplish this goal, information is routinely recorded, summarized, and monitored for trends. Such information management allows changes to be recognized and addressed promptly. Negative trends should be changed, and positive changes should be imitated or expanded. Quality improvement is focusing on what can be done for patients on an ongoing basis to achieve the desired outcomes and prevent adverse events from occurring.

There are several ways to assure the quality of care your patients receive. The major ways to be discussed in this unit are quality assurance monitoring and maintaining staff knowledge and skills.

Unit Objectives

After you successfully complete this unit, you will be able to:
- explain how quality assurance monitoring is used to assure quality patient care, and
- describe methods used to maintain staff knowledge and skills.

Unit Organization

This unit begins with a discussion of the goals of quality improvement monitoring. Methods to assure the quality of patient care and the use of outcomes measures are then described. Next, the use of this information to identify areas for improvement is explored. The unit concludes with an explanation of practices that can be used to maintain staff knowledge and skills.

Quality Assurance Monitoring

Outcomes to Measure

Before evaluating the quality of care you provide, you have to determine the desired outcomes of your services. You must select outcomes that your services are able to affect and that fall under your area of responsibility. These areas were most likely determined when you were writing a proposal or business plan for your services.

Outcomes can be general or disease specific. You may want to monitor both types. Some general outcomes include the number of hospitalizations for poor disease control or adverse effects, number of emergency room visits, utilization of other health care services, and patient satisfaction. An example of a disease-specific measure would be the percentage of patients with diabetes who achieved their target hemoglobin A_{1c}. Some example outcomes for different specialty practices are presented in **Table 1**. Disease-specific outcomes may be based on national treatment guidelines, if these exist for a particular disease. For example, the National Asthma Education Program recommends that all patients with mild persistent or worse asthma be prescribed an anti-inflammatory medication.[1]

Considerations important in selecting outcomes to measure include objectivity of a measure, ease of measuring over time (access to the information), cost of measuring over time, and consistency with standards of care. The payer of your services may also set forth expected outcomes. Health plans accredited by the National Committee on Quality Assurance (NCQA) are interested in programs that help them fulfill the standards of care set forth by NCQA, known as Healthplan Employer Data Information System (HEDIS) measures. For example, if you are in a community pharmacy setting and have a contract to provide asthma care to an insured population, you may need to track and present the following quality outcomes to the payer:
- number of hospitalizations per patient per year,
- number of emergency room visits per patient per year,
- patient satisfaction with program,
- percentage of patients performing home peak flow monitoring,
- percentage of patients using an asthma management plan, and
- percentage of patients with mild persistent or worse asthma treated with an anti-inflammatory medication.

The previously discussed quality measures look at patient outcomes of care. You may also want to examine the administrative or technical aspects of your practice. These aspects would include items such as the completeness of record notes, appropri-

Table 1. Example Disease-Specific Outcome Measures

Diabetes	% with yearly eye examination
	% meeting target HgA_{1c}
	% with annual lipid profile
Hypertension	% meeting target blood pressure goals
	% with target organ damage
Hyperlipidemia	% meeting target lipid levels
Asthma	% monitoring peak flow at home
	% utilizing an asthma management program
	number of emergency room visits for asthma exacerbations
Anticoagulation	% in target INR range
	% hospitalized for under-anticoagulation or over-anticoagulation

ate follow-up of patients who missed appointments, presence and completeness of all required forms in patient records (i.e., liability release form signed and present in chart), and quality control measures for laboratory testing.

Methods

Depending on your setting, a process to perform quality assurance monitoring may already be in place. There may even be staff devoted to such monitoring. If not, you will need to create your own methods, tracking forms, and reporting methods. Two major ways to collect information on your selected outcomes include concurrent collection and retrospective record review. With concurrent collection, you collect the necessary information at each patient visit and record this information on a data collection sheet or in a computer tracking program. You could collect concurrent information while doing patient tracking duties. Retrospective record review involves collecting the necessary information from hard copy or electronic records at a later time. Retrospective record review from hard

copy records can be difficult and time consuming, particularly if you are in a setting in which multiple health care providers use the patient records. Records may be lost or sent to another site, or the information you desire may be missing because of improper filing.

Reporting and Follow-up

The parties you need to report collected data to will vary by setting. You will at least need to review the information with all the pharmacists involved in providing services, for the purposes of continually improving those services. Data on outcomes should be reviewed to identify areas of your services that need to be improved. For example, in your anticoagulation clinic you have identified that 5% of your patients had an adverse effect with their anticoagulation therapy in the past year—a number higher than that of previous years. You can then attempt to identify the reason(s) for the increase in adverse effects and changes in clinic policies or procedures that need to be instituted. You may need to report data to your supervisors, upper management, and the payers of your services to justify and possibly expand services.

Once you have established who you need to report to and have collected data, you need to establish a mechanism for reporting the data. You can tabulate collected data by the month, quarter, year, or a combination of the three. How often you report information will be dictated by your setting and who will review the information.

Ensuring Staff Competence

Another aspect of quality care is ensuring that you and any other staff involved in providing patient care are competent to provide care and maintain up-to-date knowledge and skills. A discussion of assessing competence in patient care is beyond the scope of this book, but competence is an issue you need to consider. There are several ways for pharmacists to obtain the knowledge and skills they need to practice in a specific area and to maintain a current knowledge base. These include:

- joining specialty focused groups within the various professional organizations, sometimes called practice-related networks (PRNs) or networks;
- taking part in disease-focused education programs, including structured or continuing education programs, such as certificate programs; and
- enrolling in traineeship programs.

Traineeship programs typically provide hands-on experience in a patient care setting, whereas continuing education programs and certificate programs may only provide case-based experience and some hands-on workshop learning in physical assessment or laboratory monitoring.

Networking with peers in your local area not only helps you maintain and add to your knowledge but also provides an arena for working through problem patient cases or other practice problems. This type of networking can be accomplished by establishing a peer support group that discusses actual patient cases, recent relevant journal articles, and issues within the practice setting. The purpose of this group is to improve your medical knowledge, clinical judgment skills, and interpersonal interactions through group discussion. Sharing personal experiences fosters personal growth, an essential requirement for professionalism. Peer support groups can be especially valuable if you are in a solo practice, such as a community pharmacy setting, where you do not have other pharmacists to discuss problems and issues with.

In general, after active participation in a peer support group, members will be able to:

- develop a variety of interpersonal styles rather than maintaining the same approach for all patients,
- more comfortably handle patients/colleagues previously regarded as intolerable or frustrating, and
- facilitate the development of their clinical database and judgment skills.

Suggestions for Implementing a Peer Support Group

- Establish a meeting schedule and location that meets the needs of the majority of the participants (monthly meetings are recommended).
- Assign responsibilities, including the roles of Group Leader and Case Presenters.

Group Leader—This responsibility may be assigned to one individual or rotated among the group members. This person:

- ensures that the meeting starts on time,
- focuses on the process of discussing the case,
- proceeds to the next case presentation in an appropriate fashion, and
- encourages participants to develop multiple hypotheses and to consider a wide range of possible solutions without coming to premature closure with a plan of action for the case.

Case Presenters—Several members should be assigned the responsibility of presenting a case for discussion. The cases should be actual patients who presented a challenge to the pharmacist from a clinical and/or interpersonal perspective. All pertinent details should be presented to the group in an organized fashion. This will require preparation on the part of the presenter.

Other members are expected to contribute to the discussion to the best of their ability. They should explore all possible angles and express emotions freely.

Given the advances in electronic communications, peer support groups do not always need to be conducted face-to-face. You could set up an electronic group that posts cases and potential solutions on a Web site established for the group. With this type of arrangement, you still need a group leader to maintain control and order of the group.

Summary

Assessment of the quality of care you provide is a necessary function. When assessing quality, you need to consider what outcomes you need to measure and how to measure and report these outcomes. You also need to consider the competence of all involved staff and how competence is maintained and improved.

Reference

1.   National Institutes of Health [NIH]; National Heart, Lung, and Blood Institute. Guidelines for the diagnosis and management of asthma: National Asthma Education Program Expert Panel Report 2. Bethesda, MD: NIH; 1997. Publication No. 97–4051.

Self-Study Questions

Objective

Explain how quality assurance monitoring is used to assure quality patient care.

1. Describe how outcomes measures are chosen.

2. Which of the following does not describe outcomes measures?
    A. Outcomes measures are always disease specific.
    B. Disease-specific measures are often based on national treatment guidelines.
    C. Outcomes measures may have been previously identified in a business plan.
    D. Payers may define outcomes measures for patient care services.

3. Define concurrent and retrospective data collection.

4. Describe how outcomes measures are used to improve services.

Objective

Describe methods used to maintain staff knowledge and skills.

5. All of the following are methods for maintaining a current knowledge base *except*:
    A. membership in specialty practice groups of pharmacy associations.
    B. participation in traineeship programs.
    C. participation in peer support groups.
    D. reviewing lecture notes from pharmacy school.

6. Describe the positive impact of peer support groups.

Self-Study Answers

1. Chosen outcomes must be measurable and objective. The measures must also be something that is within your area of responsibility that you can affect. Measured outcomes can monitor patient care, administrative, and technical aspects of the pharmacy practice.

2. A

3. Concurrent data collection is when information needed for outcomes monitoring is collected and recorded in a tracking system at each patient visit. Retrospective data collection involves collecting the required information from electronic or hard copy records at a later time.

4. Outcomes measures should be analyzed for trends that indicate the need for improvement. This analysis can also show the need for new or revised policies and procedures. Outcomes with positive trends can be imitated and expanded.

5. D

6. Peer support groups may enable the care provider to develop a variety of interpersonal approaches when caring for patients, increase the ability to manage difficult providers or patients, and improve clinical knowledge and judgment skills.

Reimbursement Issues

UNIT 12

Reimbursement for patient care services is a frequently discussed topic in ambulatory care pharmacy today. Unfortunately, the majority of all pharmacy services are still reimbursed on a product rather than a service basis. The purpose of this unit is to assist you in seeking reimbursement for patient care services.

This unit assumes you will be doing your own billing. If you are in a setting where you have access to a billing department, such as a hospital-based clinic, this department will most likely do the billing for you. You need to establish a system with that department for how you will submit information specifying which services were provided to a patient. Each setting will have its own method for submitting this information.

Unit Objectives

After you successfully complete this unit, you will be able to:

- identify sources of reimbursement for patient care services,
- describe processes for obtaining reimbursement, and
- explain the impact of state and federal regulations on reimbursement.

Unit Organization

This unit begins by identifying sources of reimbursement for patient care services. Next, processes that may be successfully used to obtain reimbursement are described. The role of proper documentation in supporting reimbursement requests is also presented. The impact of state and federal regulations on reimbursement is then discussed. The unit concludes with examples of resources that may be useful in obtaining reimbursement and an example case of reimbursement in a community pharmacy setting.

Sources of Reimbursement

Some primary sources of reimbursement for ambulatory care pharmacists are cash-paying patients, traditional major medical insurance, HMOs or other health plans, integrated health systems, and, in some cases, government assistance programs such as Medicaid and Medicare.

If payment is sought at the time of service, patient payment is direct revenue. Another successful approach for some pharmacists has been to obtain reimbursement for specialized services by billing a patient's major medical insurance.

A guaranteed way to obtain reimbursement is to have a contract with a health plan, such as an HMO or integrated health system, for providing a service for a set fee (fee-for-service) or a pre-established fee (capitation). For example, you might contract with an HMO to provide asthma management services to a select group of the plan's asthma patients for $300 per patient per year.

In some instances government assistance programs are paying for pharmacist-provided patient care services, usually for pilot programs or for very specific services, such as providing immunizations. In any state, Medicare will reimburse pharmacists for providing influenza and pneumococcal pneumonia vaccinations. At this time, Mississippi has a Medicare waiver to pay pharmacists for disease management services for patients with asthma, diabetes, or hyperlipidemia and for those receiving anticoagulation therapy. The Wisconsin Medicaid program reimburses pharmacists for services that result in savings to the program.

How to Obtain Reimbursement

There are several ways to obtain reimbursement. Depending on your setting, you may choose to accept only patient out-of-pocket payment and help patients seek insurance reimbursement. This choice ensures that you are reimbursed for your services. A problem may be convincing enough patients to pay for a new or unfamiliar service, especially one with a cost attached.

For patients with traditional major medical insurance, you may choose to bill the insurance company using the procedure discussed later in this unit. You would collect unpaid amounts from the patient. Patients need to know you are billing their insurance company. They will receive a statement or explanation of benefits (EOB) from the insurance company and may question your integrity if they were not informed you were billing the insurance company. You can notify patients of your intention to bill their insurance company not only through discussion but also by having them sign a release of information statement.

If you choose to pursue a reimbursement contract with a health plan, such as an HMO, an integrated health system, or a self-insured employer, you need to identify the person within the organization to whom you may present your proposal. You may not want to discuss a new contract with pharmacy benefits employees because they often do not have money for additional programs and are primarily concerned with reducing medication costs. The medical benefits department is a better target because this department controls the money that pays for hospitalization, emergency room visits, and physician care, which are the areas of costs your services are likely to reduce. Your services may increase medication costs because you are ensuring patients actually take their medications and are on the appropriate medications. To ensure the best chance of obtaining reimbursement, seek out the party at risk for the costs of patient care impacted by your services.

With a contract for services, you will have a prearranged method for billing the payer and receiving payment. This method may involve filing individual claims or monthly or quarterly summaries of patients seen, or receiving a set amount of money no matter how many patients you see.

Before You Begin Billing

Before seeking reimbursement for your services, you need to establish a fee schedule. Fees can be charged individually (e.g., $25 per visit) or on a capitated basis. Capitation is providing all patient care, regardless of the number of visits or tests necessary, for a set fee per month or year. For example, you might provide a patient's asthma care for $300 per year.

You must charge all parties the same fees—individuals and insurers. Charging a lower fee to a patient paying out-of-pocket than what is charged to an insurance company is considered fraud. With contracts, you may negotiate fees that are different from what you normally charge individuals or insurance companies.

You also need to understand the coding systems for medical billing, necessary identification numbers, and basic forms and documents. These include current procedural terminology (CPT) codes; International Classification of Disease Ninth Revision, Clinical Modification (ICD-9-CM or, more commonly, ICD-9) codes; provider identification numbers; statements of medical necessity; and

the most commonly used claim form, the HCFA 1500.

CPT Codes

Current procedural terminology (CPT) codes explain to the payer what was done to the patient. CPT codes are created by and published annually in the *Physicians' Current Procedural Terminology* manual by the American Medical Association. These five-digit codes are used by physicians, physical therapists, chiropractors, and other allied health providers to describe medical services and procedures. The coding manual is set up in six broad categories—evaluation and management, anesthesia, surgery, radiology, pathology and laboratory, and medicine.

Selecting CPT Codes

There are codes for calls, conferences, consultation, counseling, evaluation and management, established patients, new patients, immunizations, preventive medicine, nursing facility services, second opinion, and third opinion. The codes most used by pharmacists are evaluation and management (E/M) codes for new and established patients (99201–99205 and 99211–99215, respectively) for office or outpatient visits, or for consultation. The E/M codes are determined based on the level of history taking, patient examination, medical decision-making, problem severity, coordination of care, and time spent face-to-face with the patient. The first three items are key in determining the correct code. For example, to use the 99203 code all three key components—detailed history, detailed examination, and low-complexity decision-making—must be met. If >50% of the time spent face-to-face with the patient is counseling, the code chosen can be based on time alone. **Table 1** lists E/M codes for an office or other outpatient service with a new patient.

Another aspect of CPT coding is deciding whether a patient is new or established. A new patient is one who is being seen by the provider for the first time or has not received care from the provider within 3 years. An office or outpatient visit consultation code is used when a patient is referred to the pharmacist by the physician for opinion or advice regarding evaluation and/or management of a specific problem as requested by a physician. If anything other than an opinion or advice is the result of the visit, an office or outpatient visit code should be used rather than a consultation code. For example, a patient is referred to a pharmacist for a medication review. The pharmacist reviews the patient's medications and presents recommendations

Table 1. E/M Codes for Office or Other Outpatient Services—New Patient

E/M	History	Exam	Medical Decision-Making	Problem Severity	Coordination of Care; Counseling (Average)	Time Spent Face-to-Face
99201	Problem-focused	Problem-focused	Straight-forward	Minor or self-limited	Consistent with problem(s) and patient needs	10 min.
99202	Expanded; problem-focused	Expanded; problem-focused	Straight-forward	Low to moderate	Consistent with problem(s) and patient needs	20 min.
99203	Detailed	Detailed	Low complexity	Moderate	Consistent with problem(s) and patient needs	30 min.
99204	Compre-hensive	Compre-hensive	Moderate complexity	Moderate to high	Consistent with problem(s) and patient needs	45 min.
99205	Compre-hensive	Compre-hensive	High complexity	Moderate to high	Consistent with problem(s) and patient needs	60 min.

Source: *Physicians' Current Procedural Terminology 1998.* Chicago, IL: American Medical Association; 1998.

for changes to the physician. This visit would be billed as an office or outpatient consultation visit. The code in this case would be 99241, regardless of whether it is a new or established patient. A visit where the patient was referred for diabetes education would be billed as an office or outpatient visit. In this instance, the code for a new patient is 99201 and 99211 for an established patient.

Table 2 provides a scheme for deciding on the appropriate code. The CPT manual provides additional information and criteria to help practitioners determine appropriate codes. Individual payers may want you to use a specific code for billing your services that may or may not be a CPT code.

Your documentation for each patient visit must support your choice of CPT code for billing, in case you are ever audited by an insurance company. Include in your documentation at least the key elements: patient history taken, physical examination conducted, and complexity of medical decision-making. It is preferable to include all elements.

Consider the example of a patient being referred for asthma education. This visit would be considered an office or outpatient visit. The patient has not been seen by you before, so he or she is considered a new patient. During the visit, you take a detailed medical history (including extended history of present illness; extended review of systems; and pertinent past medical, family, and social history) and conduct an expanded problem-focused physical examination (lung examination, peak flow measurement, and pulse). You have a limited amount of data to review and the patient's only health concern is asthma. This patient visit is at a low level of complexity of decision-making. You spend 30 minutes with the patient, of which 20 minutes is counseling time. In this case, because >50% of your time face-to-face with the patient was spent counseling, time becomes the determining factor in selecting a CPT code. You would use the 99203 code.

ICD-9 Codes

International Classification of Disease Ninth Revision (ICD-9) codes are used by most payers to classify the diagnoses, conditions, problems, or other reasons for an encounter with health care professionals. ICD-9 codes are diagnosis codes assigned by a physician or other health professional allowed by law to diagnose. The codes are at least three digits long, with some codes having up to five digits. The last two digits are for increasing specificity.

Medicare requires the use of ICD-9 codes at their highest level of specificity, which means you must use a fourth or fifth digit when one exists. For example, the shortened code for asthma is 493.9, whereas more specific codes are 493.90 (asthma without status asthmaticus) and 493.91 (asthma with status asthmaticus). Medicare would reject the claim unless the five-digit code is used. Other payers may also require this level of specificity.

Obtaining ICD-9 Codes

ICD-9 codes are published in book format, but you would rarely need to consult it. It is beyond the scope of pharmacy practice to diagnose or assign a code for a patient. You must obtain the ICD-9 code from the patient's physician and bill under the same code as the physician to avoid any indication of fraud. You can obtain the correct ICD-9 code by requesting this information on a statement of medical necessity (discussed later) or by calling the referring physician's billing office. Always document the source of the code you are using for a particular patient.

Provider Identification Numbers

These numbers identify providers to the health care payer. Physicians have a universal provider identification number (UPIN), national provider identifier (NPI), or provider identification number (PIN). For physicians, the system for assigning identification numbers is moving to NPI numbers only but is currently in transition, so a physician might use all three numbers. If you need the physician's identification number for billing, you can request this information on a statement of medical necessity or you can call the referring physician's office. Depending on the payer being billed, pharmacists may or may not need provider numbers.

How to Obtain a Provider Number

When billing some health plans, you need to have a provider number that identifies you to the billing department of the plan. Some plans accept a Medicare provider number, but others require an individual provider number. If you have a contract for service with a plan, you can arrange in advance what provider information you are to provide on billing forms. If you are billing a major medical insurance plan, you need to contact the plan to find out how to obtain a provider number and how they would like you to bill for services.

At this time, pharmacies can obtain a provider number from Medicare, but this number is only good for billing for immunizations or supplying

Table 2. Choosing a CPT Code

1. Is patient new or established?
   __ new
   __ established
   (*new*—seen by provider for the first time or has not received professional care from provider or another provider of the same specialty group within 3 years)

2. What category or subcategory of E/M service is this?
   __ office or other outpatient service
   __ office or outpatient consultation
   __ case management service
      __ team conference
      __ telephone call
   __ preventive medicine services
      __ evaluation and management
      __ individual counseling
      __ group counseling

3. Extent of history obtained:
   __ problem focused (brief history of present illness [HPI], no review of systems [ROS], no past/family/social history [PFSH])
   __ expanded problem focused (brief HPI, problem-pertinent ROS, no PFSH)
   __ detailed (extended HPI, extended ROS, pertinent PFSH)
   __ comprehensive (extended HPI, complete ROS, complete PFSH)

4. Extent of examination of patient:
   __ problem focused (limited examination of affected body area or organ system)
   __ expanded problem focused (limited examination of affected body area or organ system and any other symptomatic or related body area[s] or organ system[s])
   __ detailed (extended examination of affected body area or organ system and any other symptomatic or related body area[s] or organ system[s])
   __ comprehensive (general multisystem or complete examination of a single organ system or other symptomatic or related body area[s] or organ system[s])

5. Complexity of decision-making:
   __ straightforward (minimal number of diag-

noses or management options, minimal or no amount and/or complexity of data to be reviewed, minimal risk of complications and/or morbidity and/or mortality)
   __ low complexity (limited number of diagnoses or management options, limited amount and/or complexity of data to be reviewed, low risk of complications and/or morbidity and/or mortality)
   __ moderate complexity (multiple number of diagnoses or management options, moderate amount and/or complexity of data to be reviewed, moderate risk of complications and/or morbidity and/or mortality)
   __ high complexity (extensive number of diagnoses or management options, extensive amount and/or complexity of data to be reviewed, high risk of complications and/or morbidity and/or mortality)
   (two of the three elements must be met or exceeded to justify level)

6. Which topics was patient counseled on?
   __ risks and benefits of treatment options
   __ instructions for management and/or follow-up
   __ importance of compliance with treatment
   __ risk factor reduction
   __ patient education
   __ family education

7. What coordination of care was provided?
   __ coordinated with other providers/agencies with a patient visit on that day
   __ coordinated with other providers/agencies without a patient visit on that day

8. Which is the nature of the presenting problem?
   __ minimal (problem may not require the presence of the provider but service is rendered under provider's supervision)
   __ self-limited or minor (problem runs a definite and prescribed course, is transient in nature and is not likely to permanently alter health status, or has a good prognosis with management/compliance)
   __ low severity (problem in which the risk of morbidity without treatment is low, there is little to no risk of mortality without treat-

ment, and/or full recovery without functional impairment is expected)

__ moderate severity (problem where the risk of morbidity without treatment is moderate, there is moderate risk of mortality without treatment, and/or uncertain prognosis or increased probability of prolonged functional impairment)

__ high severity (problem where the risk of morbidity without treatment is high to extreme; there is moderate to high risk of mortality without treatment; and/or high probability of severe, prolonged functional impairment)

9. How much time was spent face-to-face with the patient?

_____

The reader is advised to consult the CPT manual for further explanation of all terms.

Source: *Physicians' Current Procedural Terminology 1998*. Chicago, IL: American Medical Association; 1998, and *Coding and Reimbursement Guide for Pharmacists*. Reston, VA: St. Anthony Publishing; 1997.

Table 3. Questions to Ask a Health Plan Billing Department

- Will the plan cover pharmaceutical care services?
- Is a physician referral or preauthorization necessary (completion of a statement of medical necessity)?
- Is preauthorization from the plan necessary?
- Is there a maximum number of visits allowed per year?
- Which claim forms must be used?
- How can claims be sent?
- Are there any payer-specific codes that must be used?
- Is a provider identification number required?
- How does one obtain a provider identification number?

durable medical equipment (DME). To obtain a Medicare provider number, contact the Medicare carrier for your state or region, request the Medicare Provider/Suppler Enrollment Application (HCFA-855 form), fill out the appropriate sections of the application (Mass Immunizer or DME Supplier sections), and return it to the carrier.

Statement of Medical Necessity

A statement of medical necessity is essentially a referral form from a physician stating that it is medically necessary for a patient to receive your services. This statement should outline what services you are to provide to the patient (an example appears in **Figure 1**). This statement may or may not be required by a payer.

HCFA 1500 Claim Form

The HCFA 1500 claim form is a nationally standardized form developed by the Health Care Financing Administration (HCFA) to report services provided by most health care professionals (an example of the form appears in **Figure 2**). This is the claim form accepted by most health care payers. HCFA 1500 claim forms may be obtained from office supply stores, medical supply catalogs, and billing software companies.

When billing using a form such as the HCFA 1500, you will need to use appropriate CPT codes to explain to the payer what services were performed for the patients and ICD-9 codes to identify the patients' problems or reason for visit, unless directed to do otherwise by the payer. A physician identification number is usually needed if a physician has referred a patient to you for services. Under contract billing, you may or may not need these codes and numbers.

How to Bill

To increase your likelihood of being paid you should contact the plan you will be billing to determine the procedure to be followed. The patient's insurance card will usually have a telephone number you can call to obtain information as a provider. Some questions to ask are included in **Table 3**.

Once you have the specific information for an individual plan, you can then complete the forms required by the plan (usually the HCFA 1500). The form must be filled out correctly and completely for a payer to process the claim.

The steps to filling out the HCFA 1500 form are outlined below. The numbers given refer to the

STATEMENT OF MEDICAL NECESSITY

Patient Name: _____   Date:_____

Address: _____

City: _____ State:_____ Zip: _____

Home Telephone:_____ Date of Birth: _____

Diagnosis (ICD-9) _____

Patient Problem(s): _____

_____

Requested Services   (✓)

• Comprehensive _____ self-management instruction   _____

• Self-management assessment   _____

• Home monitoring instruction

        • _____   _____

        • _____   _____

• Medication administration instruction (_____)   _____

• Medication regimen adherence   _____

Goals of service requested: _____

_____

Anticipated duration:_____

I consider these requested services to be a necessary part of the patient's care.

_____   _____

Physician's Signature   *Date*

Physician Name (print): _____

Practice Address: _____

Telephone: _____ UPIN/NPI: _____

Figure 1. Statement of Medical Necessity

Figure 2. HCFA 1500 Claim Form

numbered spaces on the form (see **Figure 2**). Spaces 1–13 request patient information and insured information and are self-explanatory, with a few exceptions. In space 4, enter the name of the insured only when that person's insurance is primary to Medicare. If Medicare is primary, leave the space blank. If the insured and the patient are the same person, enter "same." Spaces 9–9d are used for information on Medigap policies, which cover what Medicare does not pay. Pharmacists do not use these spaces. Space 11d should be left blank; it is not required by most third-party payers. The patient does not have to physically sign space 12 if you have a signed authorization form on file to bill the patient's insurance (part of the patient release statement, discussed in unit 10). In this case, you can enter "SOF" for "signature on file."

Spaces 13–33 request information on the service provided to the patient and the supplier of the service's information. Again, many of the items are self-explanatory. Spaces 17 and 17a must be completed if the patient was referred by a physician. Space 21 is for the ICD-9 codes that specify the diagnoses, conditions, problems, or other reasons for the encounter. At least one code must be reported.

A complete listing of place of service codes for space 24b is available from your regional Medicare carrier or the *Coding and Reimbursement Guide for Pharmacists* (noted in **Table 4**). Here are some example codes that might be used by pharmacists:

    11 Doctor's office
    60 Mass immunization site
    72 Rural health clinic
    71 State or local public health clinic
    99 Other unlisted facility

An example completed HCFA 1500 can be found in **Figure 3**. Once the HCFA 1500 is completed, mail it to the appropriate address for the payer with any other documentation required by the payer or that you feel will support your claim for reimbursement. The mailing address should be listed on the patient's insurance card. Although many payers accept electronic claim submission, you cannot submit additional documentation with an electronic claim. Most pharmacists submit claims manually because additional documentation is being included. **Table 5** outlines the steps in the billing process.

Table 4. Coding, Terminology, and Reimbursement Resources

Coding and Reimbursement Guide for Pharmacists (book) and "Payment Strategies for Pharmaceutical Care" (monthly newsletter)
St. Anthony Publishing and the American Pharmaceutical Association
11410 Isaac Newton Square
Reston, VA 20190
(703) 904-3900

Physician's Current Procedural Terminology (published yearly, standard and professional editions, and companion for training and reference)
American Medical Association
P.O. Box 7046
Dover, DE 19903-7046
(800) 621-8335
www.ama-assn.org

Table 5. Billing Steps

Initially:
1. Obtain a supplier/provider number.
2. Obtain HCFA 1500 or other appropriate claim forms.
3. Establish fees.

For each patient:
1. Obtain patient insurance and medical diagnosis information (ICD-9 code).
2. Contact insurer for patient to determine procedure for billing, if not already done.
3. Obtain statement of medical necessity, if necessary.
4. Select appropriate CPT code.
5. Complete HCFA 1500 and attach any supporting documentation.
6. Submit to insurer.
7. Follow up by tracking paid and rejected claims.
8. Resubmit rejected claims with any errors corrected.

PLEASE
DO NOT
STAPLE
IN THIS
AREA

HEALTH INSURANCE CLAIM FORM

☐☐ PICA   PICA ☐☐

1. MEDICARE	MEDICAID	CHAMPUS	CHAMPVA	GROUP HEALTH PLAN	FECA BLK LUNG	OTHER	1a. INSURED'S I.D. NUMBER (FOR PROGRAM IN ITEM 1)
☐ (Medicare #)	☐ (Medicaid #)	☐ (Sponsor's SSN)	☐ (VA File #)	☒ (SSN or ID)	☐ (SSN)	☐ (ID)	475869-079685

2. PATIENT'S NAME (Last Name, First Name, Middle Initial)	3. PATIENT'S BIRTH DATE SEX	4. INSURED'S NAME (Last Name, First Name, Middle Initial)
Jones, Fred	MM 06 DD 08 YY 48 M ☒ F ☐	Jones, Fred

5. PATIENT'S ADDRESS (No., Street)	6. PATIENT RELATIONSHIP TO INSURED	7. INSURED'S ADDRESS (No., Street)
1567 South Lake Blvd	Self ☒ Spouse ☐ Child ☐ Other ☐	same

CITY	STATE	8. PATIENT STATUS	CITY	STATE
Memphis	TN	Single ☐ Married ☒ Other ☐		

ZIP CODE	TELEPHONE (Include Area Code)		ZIP CODE	TELEPHONE (INCLUDE AREA CODE)
34567	(450) 345-9876	Employed ☐ Full-Time Student ☐ Part-Time Student ☐		( )

9. OTHER INSURED'S NAME (Last Name, First Name, Middle Initial)	10. IS PATIENT'S CONDITION RELATED TO:	11. INSURED'S POLICY GROUP OR FECA NUMBER

a. OTHER INSURED'S POLICY OR GROUP NUMBER	a. EMPLOYMENT? (CURRENT OR PREVIOUS) ☐ YES ☐ NO	a. INSURED'S DATE OF BIRTH MM 06 DD 08 YY 48 SEX M ☒ F ☐

b. OTHER INSURED'S DATE OF BIRTH SEX MM DD YY M ☐ F ☐	b. AUTO ACCIDENT? PLACE (State) ☐ YES ☐ NO	b. EMPLOYER'S NAME OR SCHOOL NAME Alameda School Board

c. EMPLOYER'S NAME OR SCHOOL NAME	c. OTHER ACCIDENT? ☐ YES ☐ NO	c. INSURANCE PLAN NAME OR PROGRAM NAME Southern Insurance Company

d. INSURANCE PLAN NAME OR PROGRAM NAME	10d. RESERVED FOR LOCAL USE	d. IS THERE ANOTHER HEALTH BENEFIT PLAN? ☐ YES ☒ NO If yes, return to and complete item 9 a-d.

READ BACK OF FORM BEFORE COMPLETING & SIGNING THIS FORM.

12. PATIENT'S OR AUTHORIZED PERSON'S SIGNATURE I authorize the release of any medical or other information necessary to process this claim. I also request payment of government benefits either to myself or to the party who accepts assignment below.

SIGNED   Signature on File   DATE   04/08/99

13. INSURED'S OR AUTHORIZED PERSON'S SIGNATURE I authorize payment of medical benefits to the undersigned physician or supplier for services described below.

SIGNED   Signature on File

14. DATE OF CURRENT: ◄ ILLNESS (First symptom) OR INJURY (Accident) OR PREGNANCY(LMP) MM DD YY	15. IF PATIENT HAS HAD SAME OR SIMILAR ILLNESS. GIVE FIRST DATE MM DD YY	16. DATES PATIENT UNABLE TO WORK IN CURRENT OCCUPATION MM DD YY FROM TO MM DD YY

17. NAME OF REFERRING PHYSICIAN OR OTHER SOURCE Lewis, Robert	17a. I.D. NUMBER OF REFERRING PHYSICIAN S57849	18. HOSPITALIZATION DATES RELATED TO CURRENT SERVICES MM DD YY FROM TO MM DD YY

19. RESERVED FOR LOCAL USE	20. OUTSIDE LAB? $ CHARGES ☐ YES ☐ NO

21. DIAGNOSIS OR NATURE OF ILLNESS OR INJURY. (RELATE ITEMS 1,2,3 OR 4 TO ITEM 24E BY LINE)	22. MEDICAID RESUBMISSION CODE ORIGINAL REF. NO.
1. 250.00 3.	23. PRIOR AUTHORIZATION NUMBER
2. 4.	

24. A. DATE(S) OF SERVICE					B. Place of Service	C. Type of Service	D. PROCEDURES, SERVICES, OR SUPPLIES (Explain Unusual Circumstances) CPT/HCPCS	MODIFIER	E. DIAGNOSIS CODE	F. $ CHARGES	G. DAYS OR UNITS	H. EPSDT Family Plan	I. EMG	J. COB	K. RESERVED FOR LOCAL USE
From MM DD YY		To MM DD YY													
04 08 99	04 08 99	99					99213		1	45 00	1				

25. FEDERAL TAX I.D. NUMBER SSN EIN 95-3772572 ☒	26. PATIENT'S ACCOUNT NO.	27. ACCEPT ASSIGNMENT? (For govt. claims, see back) ☒ YES ☐ NO	28. TOTAL CHARGE $ 45 00	29. AMOUNT PAID $ 0 00	30. BALANCE DUE $ 45 00

31. SIGNATURE OF PHYSICIAN OR SUPPLIER INCLUDING DEGREES OR CREDENTIALS (I certify that the statements on the reverse apply to this bill and are made a part thereof.)	32. NAME AND ADDRESS OF FACILITY WHERE SERVICES WERE RENDERED (If other than home or office)	33. PHYSICIAN'S, SUPPLIER'S BILLING NAME, ADDRESS, ZIP CODE & PHONE #
Joe Smith, R.Ph SIGNED 04/08/99 DATE		Specialty Pharmacy 1400 East Main Street Memphis, TN 34567
		PIN# 576890 GRP#

(APPROVED BY AMA COUNCIL ON MEDICAL SERVICE 8/88)   **PLEASE PRINT OR TYPE**

FORM HCFA-1500 (12-90)
FORM OWCP-1500   FORM RRB-1500

Figure 3. Completed HCFA 1500 Claim Form

Billing Documentation

You need to maintain documentation to support your billing efforts. Some of the documents you need to maintain (as applicable) are patient notes; statement or certificate of medical necessity; preauthorization information from the health care payer; copies of any pertinent legislative, regulatory, or certification paperwork; patient release of information statements; and your rationale for selecting the specific CPT codes.

Patient notes should provide some of the elements necessary in documenting your choice of CPT codes, including history obtained, examination completed, counseling completed with patient or family, and time spent with the patient. Maintain copies of any legislation or regulation that allows you to bill for services. It may expedite payment of claims to include a copy of this legislation or regulation with your claim forms. For example, pharmacists in New Jersey who have completed appropriate training programs are able to bill for diabetes self-management education. These pharmacists may include a copy of the law when submitting a claim.

Some pharmacists include a cover letter to the payer with their claim submissions. A cover letter can clarify for the payer that the service was provided by a pharmacist and not a physician. An example of a cover letter can be found in **Figure 4**.

State and Federal Guidelines for Reimbursement

As discussed at the beginning of this unit, you must be aware of your state laws that relate to reimbursement. At this time, the federal government does not reimburse pharmacists for providing pharmaceutical care except where individual states have Medicare waivers for specific projects. There are currently no federal guidelines for reimbursing pharmacists, but this may change. Because of the changing nature of this topic, the reader is advised to stay up-to-date with state and federal regulations regarding pharmacist reimbursement.

Reimbursement Resources

Some resources for additional information are the reimbursement specialists or billing department within your setting, billing companies, professional organizations (especially specialty interest groups within the organization who may be confronting the same issues as you), and publishing companies, such as St. Anthony Publishing. **Table 4** lists some print resources for reimbursement.

Billing software is available for completing claims. Initially, you can fill out the claim form by hand. Once you are submitting a larger number of claim forms, you may wish to invest in billing software such as Just Claims. Some pharmacy dispensing software will also complete HCFA 1500 claim forms.

Case Study

Roark's Pharmacy is a community pharmacy located in Oneida, a rural community in eastern Tennessee. The pharmacy has two full-time pharmacists, a husband and wife team, Terry and Mary Anne Roark. They have an average prescription volume of 250 per day. Currently they offer an asthma management service and plan to expand to include a diabetes management service. Patients with asthma are seen on slower days in the middle of the week. Mary Anne receives referrals from area physicians (**Figure 5**). She charges patients $85 for up to three visits (an initial visit and two follow-up consultations, if necessary). Because reimbursement has been limited from private insurers, patients pay up front and are provided with the necessary forms to submit claims to their insurance company. **Figure 6** shows a form letter the patient is given with a completed HCFA 1500 (**Figure 7**) and a copy of the physician referral. According to the Roarks, the patients receive reimbursement from their insurance company about 10% of the time.

The majority of the time the patients receive an explanation of benefits (EOB) stating that the service is not a covered benefit. When patients have been reimbursed, they have received $60–75.

Summary

Reimbursement for providing pharmaceutical care is in its infancy. This unit has presented information on potential sources of reimbursement and how to begin submitting bills to insurance companies. Because there is no set way to obtain reimbursement, numerous strategies may need to be tried before you are successful.

Specialized Pharmacy

Tel (804) 555-1234
Fax (804) 555-5678

May 8, 1999

Diabetes Care Payer
1 Plaza Drive
Richmond, VA 23335

Dear _____:

I am requesting payment for diabetes care service provided by The Pharmacy Care Center at Specialized Pharmacy as summarized below:

PatientName: _____

Patient Address: _____

Plan Name/ID Number: _____

Date of Service: _____

Expected Outcomes: _____

_____

_____

Supporting documents enclosed:

HFCA1500 CLAIM FORM
MEDICAL NECESSITY FORM

Please submit payment to:

SPECIALIZED PHARMACY
123 MAIN STREET
RICHMOND, VIRGINIA 23333-0123

Tax ID number: 123454656

Sincerely,

Susanne Stevens, R.Ph.

Figure 4. Sample cover letter

ROARK'S PHARMACY / HOMEBIOTICS

PHYSICIAN PRESCRIPTION FOR ASTHMA MANAGEMENT REFERRAL

PATIENT'S NAME:_____   DATE: _____

PATIENT'S ADDRESS:_____   PHONE: _____

BIRTH DATE:_____ SEX: M/F   HEIGHT:_____WEIGHT _____

INSURANCE PROVIDER:_____   ID#:   _____

PATIENT DIAGNOSIS: _____

PATIENT PROGNOSIS: _____

ASTHMA SEVERITY: _____MILD _____MODERATE _____SEVERE

MEDICAL HISTORY:

___ASTHMA   ___CHRONIC BRONCHITIS ___EPILEPSY   ___KIDNEY DISEASE   ___OTHER

___CANCER   ___COPD   ___GLAUCOMA   ___LIVER DISEASE   _____

___CARDIAC   ___EAR INFECTIONS   ___HAY FEVER   ___THYROID

___CHF   ___EMPHYSEMA   ___HYPERTENSION

MEDICATION ALLERGIES: _____

CURRENT MEDICATIONS: _____

(Name, strength, frequency)_____

(Rx and OTC)   _____

                        _____

                        _____

                        _____

PREVIOUS LAB LEVELS: _____

(Theophylline mcg/ml & date) _____

BASELINE PEAK FLOW METER READING: _____

THIS PRESCRIPTION MUST BE RENEWED EVERY 12 MONTHS

PHYSICIAN'S NAME: _____

ADDRESS: _____

         _____

PHONE#: _____

FAX PH #: _____

PHYSICIAN'S U.P.I.N. NUMBER: _____

PHYSICIAN'S SIGNATURE: _____

DATE SIGNED: _____

Roark's Pharmacy   HomeBiotics
19118 Alberta Street   19118 Alberta Street
Oneida, TN 37841   Oneida, TN 37841
423-569-9000   423-569-2400
FAX 423-569-2402   FAX 423-569-2402

Figure 5. Roark's Pharmacy Referral Form

ROARK'S PHARMACY / HOMEBIOTICS
Asthma Care Center
19118 Alberta Street
Oneida, TN 37841
423-569-9000

Welcome to Roark's Pharmacy/HomeBiotics Asthma Care Center!

The staff at Roark's Pharmacy looks forward to helping patients with asthma. Our Asthma Care Program is designed to help educate the patient with information about asthma. By educating patients about proper medication administration and learning to assess and monitor the severity of the disease, patients with asthma can increase their quality of life. Management plans and individualized treatment plans will be provided to help the physician, patient, and pharmacist achieve the goals of the Asthma Care Program.

The goals of the Asthma Care Program are:
1. Improve medication skills.
2. Avoid asthma triggers.
3. Cope with the bad days. Use of a peak flow meter to monitor pulmonary function.
4. Improve on medication use patterns.
5. Work with patient and physician to establish and implement an individualized asthma action plan.

Patients are asked to pay for initial and follow-up visits on completion of each appointment. An itemized bill of services rendered will be provided for each patient.

We think that our Asthma Care Program will help patients feel better and live longer. Please contact us if you or a family member have any questions or concerns.

Roark's Pharmacy
Terry and Mary Anne Roark, pharmacists
19118 Alberta Street
Oneida, TN 37841
423-569-9000
FAX 423-569-2402

Figure 6. Roark's Pharmacy form letter

PLEASE
DO NOT
STAPLE
IN THIS
AREA

| | PICA | | **HEALTH INSURANCE CLAIM FORM** | PICA | |

| 1. MEDICARE (Medicare #) | MEDICAID (Medicaid #) | CHAMPUS (Sponsor's SSN) | CHAMPVA (VA File #) | GROUP HEALTH PLAN (SSN or ID) | FECA BLK LUNG (SSN) | OTHER [X] (ID) | 1a. INSURED'S I.D. NUMBER (FOR PROGRAM IN ITEM 1) XTZ 410876543 |

2. PATIENT'S NAME (Last Name, First Name, Middle Initial)
Smith, Jane

3. PATIENT'S BIRTH DATE MM DD YY 02 17 55   SEX M [ ] F [X]

4. INSURED'S NAME (Last Name, First Name, Middle Initial)
Smith, Jane

5. PATIENT'S ADDRESS (No., Street)
415 S. Main St.

6. PATIENT RELATIONSHIP TO INSURED
Self [X] Spouse [ ] Child [ ] Other [ ]

7. INSURED'S ADDRESS (No., Street)
same

CITY **Oneida**   STATE **TN**

8. PATIENT STATUS
Single [ ] Married [X] Other [ ]

CITY   STATE

ZIP CODE **37841**   TELEPHONE (Include Area Code) **(423) 569-1234**

Employed [ ] Full-Time Student [X] Part-Time Student [ ]

ZIP CODE   TELEPHONE (INCLUDE AREA CODE) ( )

9. OTHER INSURED'S NAME (Last Name, First Name, Middle Initial)

10. IS PATIENT'S CONDITION RELATED TO:

11. INSURED'S POLICY GROUP OR FECA NUMBER

a. OTHER INSURED'S POLICY OR GROUP NUMBER

a. EMPLOYMENT? (CURRENT OR PREVIOUS) YES [ ] NO [X]

a. INSURED'S DATE OF BIRTH MM DD YY 02 17 55   SEX M [ ] F [X]

b. OTHER INSURED'S DATE OF BIRTH MM DD YY   SEX M [ ] F [ ]

b. AUTO ACCIDENT? PLACE (State) YES [ ] NO [X]

b. EMPLOYER'S NAME OR SCHOOL NAME
Pinaco Flooring

c. EMPLOYER'S NAME OR SCHOOL NAME

c. OTHER ACCIDENT? YES [ ] NO [ ]

c. INSURANCE PLAN NAME OR PROGRAM NAME
American Standard Ins. Co.

d. INSURANCE PLAN NAME OR PROGRAM NAME

10d. RESERVED FOR LOCAL USE

d. IS THERE ANOTHER HEALTH BENEFIT PLAN?
YES [ ] NO [X]   If yes, return to and complete item 9 a-d.

READ BACK OF FORM BEFORE COMPLETING & SIGNING THIS FORM.

12. PATIENT'S OR AUTHORIZED PERSON'S SIGNATURE I authorize the release of any medical or other information necessary to process this claim. I also request payment of government benefits either to myself or to the party who accepts assignment below.

SIGNED *Jane Smith*   DATE **9-3-98**

13. INSURED'S OR AUTHORIZED PERSON'S SIGNATURE I authorize payment of medical benefits to the undersigned physician or supplier for services described below.

SIGNED *Jane Smith*

14. DATE OF CURRENT: ILLNESS (First symptom) OR INJURY (Accident) OR PREGNANCY(LMP) MM DD YY 08 12 98

15. IF PATIENT HAS HAD SAME OR SIMILAR ILLNESS. GIVE FIRST DATE MM DD YY 01 15 98

16. DATES PATIENT UNABLE TO WORK IN CURRENT OCCUPATION FROM 08 12 98 TO 08 20 98

17. NAME OF REFERRING PHYSICIAN OR OTHER SOURCE
Dr. Jones

17a. I.D. NUMBER OF REFERRING PHYSICIAN
U.P.I.N.#

18. HOSPITALIZATION DATES RELATED TO CURRENT SERVICES FROM 08 15 98 TO 08 16 98

19. RESERVED FOR LOCAL USE

20. OUTSIDE LAB? YES [ ] NO [X] $ CHARGES

21. DIAGNOSIS OR NATURE OF ILLNESS OR INJURY. (RELATE ITEMS 1,2,3 OR 4 TO ITEM 24E BY LINE)
1. **493.20**
2. ___.___
3. ___.___
4. ___.___

22. MEDICAID RESUBMISSION CODE   ORIGINAL REF. NO.

23. PRIOR AUTHORIZATION NUMBER

24. A DATE(S) OF SERVICE			B Place of Service	C Type of Service	D PROCEDURES, SERVICES, OR SUPPLIES (Explain Unusual Circumstances) CPT/HCPCS MODIFIER	E DIAGNOSIS CODE	F $ CHARGES	G DAYS OR UNITS	H EPSDT Family Plan	I EMG	J COB	K RESERVED FOR LOCAL USE
From MM DD YY	To MM DD YY											
09 03 98	09 03 98		99		99213	1	85 00	1				

25. FEDERAL TAX I.D. NUMBER SSN EIN
62-1234567 [X]

26. PATIENT'S ACCOUNT NO.

27. ACCEPT ASSIGNMENT? (For govt. claims, see back) YES [ ] NO [X]

28. TOTAL CHARGE $ **85 00**

29. AMOUNT PAID $

30. BALANCE DUE $

31. SIGNATURE OF PHYSICIAN OR SUPPLIER INCLUDING DEGREES OR CREDENTIALS (I certify that the statements on the reverse apply to this bill and are made a part thereof.)

SIGNED **9-3-98**

32. NAME AND ADDRESS OF FACILITY WHERE SERVICES WERE RENDERED (If other than home or office)

33. PHYSICIAN'S, SUPPLIER'S BILLING NAME, ADDRESS, ZIP CODE & PHONE #
Roark's Pharmacy 423-569-9009
19118 Alberta St.
Oneida, TN 37841
PIN#   GRP#

(APPROVED BY AMA COUNCIL ON MEDICAL SERVICE 8/88)   **PLEASE PRINT OR TYPE**   FORM HCFA-1500 (12-90) FORM OWCP-1500   FORM RRB-1500

Figure 7. Completed HCFA 1500 submitted by Roark's Pharmacy

Self-Study Questions

Objective
Identify sources of reimbursement for patient care services.

1. List potential sources of reimbursement for patient care services.

Objective
Describe processes for obtaining reimbursement.

2. Which of the following is not a process for obtaining reimbursement for patient care services?

    A. billing the Department of Health and Human Services for patients covered by Medicare

    B. collecting payment from the patient at the time the service is provided

    C. contracting with a health plan to provide services for patients covered by the plan

    D. billing the patient's medical insurance and collecting unpaid amounts from the patient

3. Describe how fees for services are established.

4. What are the primary determinants of a CPT code?

5. When choosing a CPT code, what is the difference between a new and established patient?

6. Which of the following is not usually done by the pharmacist?

    A. assigning a CPT code

    B. assigning an ICD-9 code

    C. obtaining a Medicare provider number

    D. filing an HCFA 1500 claim form

7. Describe the importance of documentation in obtaining reimbursement and give examples of documentation.

Objective
Explain the impact of state and federal regulations on reimbursement.

8. Describe current state and federal regulations for reimbursement.

Self-Study Answers

1. Cash-paying patients, major medical insurance providers, health care plans, integrated health care systems, and government assistance programs are all potential sources of reimbursement.

2. A

3. Fees may be set for an individual service or capitated for all services provided to a patient or group of a patients. When establishing fees, it is important to charge the same fee to individuals as well as insurers to avoid charges of fraud. One exception is contracted services, in which case a lower charge for a service may be negotiated.

4. The primary components that determine a CPT code are the level of patient history taking, the extent of physical examination, and the complexity of decision-making.

5. A new patient is one who is being seen for the first time or one who has not been seen for more than 3 years. An established patient is one who is not described by these criteria.

6. B

7. Documentation that supports your claim for reimbursement should be provided. Examples include patient notes, referral letters, statements of medical necessity, copies of legislation and regulations that allow you to bill for services, and patient release of information forms.

8. At the present time, there are no federal guidelines for reimbursement for pharmacy services. However, there are several states in which pilot programs have been established for reimbursement of services provided to Medicare patients.

APPENDIXES

Blank Forms

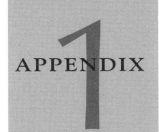

APPENDIX 1

DEPARTMENT OF HEALTH AND HUMAN SERVICES
HEALTH CARE FINANCING ADMINISTRATION

FORM APPROVED
OMB NO. 0938-0581

CLINICAL LABORATORY APPLICATION
CLINICAL LABORATORY IMPROVEMENT AMENDMENTS OF 1988

Public reporting burden for this collection of information is estimated to vary between 30 minutes to 2 hours per response , including time for reviewing instructions, searching existing data sources, gathering and maintaining data needed, and completing and reviewing the collection of information. Send any comments including suggestions for reducing the burden to the Office of Financial Management, HCFA, P.O. Box 26684, Baltimore, MD 21207; and to the Office of Management and Budget, Paperwork Reduction Project (0938-0581), Washington, D.C. 20503.

I. GENERAL INFORMATION

Please check any preprinted information on this part of the form and make any necessary corrections. Complete the rest of the form according to the directions.

CLIA IDENTIFICATION NUMBER	FEDERAL TAX IDENTIFICATION NUMBER		
LABORATORY NAME	TELEPHONE NO. *(include area code)*		
LABORATORY ADDRESS *(number, street)*	CITY	STATE	ZIP
MAILING ADDRESS *(if different from above)*	CITY	STATE	ZIP

NAME OF DIRECTOR *(please print or type)*

last   first   MI

Indicate changes below as needed.

LABORATORY NAME	TELEPHONE NO. *(include area code)*		
LABORATORY ADDRESS *(number, street)*	CITY	STATE	ZIP
MAILING ADDRESS *(if different from above)*	CITY	STATE	ZIP

NAME OF DIRECTOR *(please print or type)*

last   first   MI

II. APPLICATION IS FOR: *(check one box)*

☐ Certificate   ☐ Renewal of Certificate
☐ **Certificate of Waiver   ☐ Renewal of Certificate of Waiver
☐ Certificate of Accreditation   ☐ Renewal of Certificate of Accreditation

**IF YOU CONDUCT ONLY THE FOLLOWING WAIVED TESTS *(ONE OR MORE)*, YOU MAY APPLY FOR A CERTIFICATE OF WAIVER:.

•Dipstick or tablet reagent urinalysis (nonautomated) for:

-bilirubin	-glucose
-hemoglobin	-ketone
-leukocytes	-nitrite
-protein	-pH
-specific gravity	-urobilinogen

•Fecal occult blood
•Ovulation test-visual color comparison tests for human luteinizing hormone

•Urine pregnancy test-visual color comparison tests
•Erythrocyte sedimentation rate (nonautomated)
•Hemoglobin-copper sulfate (nonautomated)
•Blood glucose, by glucose monitoring devices cleared by the FDA specifically for home use; and
•Spun microhematocrit

If applying for a **certificate of waiver,** complete all sections of this form except section VIII.

FORM HCFA-116 (8-92)   Page 1 of 4

Health Care Financing Agency (HCFA) Form 116

III. TYPE OF LABORATORY *(check the __one__ most descriptive of facility type)*

___ 01 Ambulatory Surgery Center
___ 02 Community Clinic
___ 03 Comp. Outpatient Rehab. Facility
___ 04 Ancillary Testing Site in Health Care Facility
___ 05 End Stage Renal Disease Dialysis Facility
___ 06 Health Fair
___ 07 Health Main. Organization

___ 08 Home Health Agency
___ 09 Hospice
___ 10 Hospital
___ 11 Independent
___ 12 Industrial
___ 13 Insurance
___ 14 Intermediate Care Fac. for Mentally Retarded

___ 15 Mobile Unit
___ 16 Pharmacy
___ 17 School/Student Health Service
___ 18 Skilled Nursing Facility/Nursing Facility
___ 19 Physician Office
___ 20 Other Practitioner *(specify)* _____
___ 21 Tissue Bank/Repositories
___ 22 Blood Banks
___ 23 Other *(specify)* _____

Was this __laboratory__ previously regulated under the Federal Medicare/Medicaid and/or CLIA programs? (Regulations published March 14, 1990 at 55 FR 9538) .... ☐ Yes   ☐ No

IV. HOURS OF ROUTINE OPERATION

List days and hours during which __laboratory testing__ is performed

	SUNDAY	MONDAY	TUESDAY	WEDNESDAY	THURSDAY	FRIDAY	SATURDAY
FROM: AM							
PM							
TO: AM							
PM							

(For multiple sites attach the additional information using the same format)

V. MULTIPLE SITES

Are you applying for one certificate for multiple sites?   ☐ No *If no,* go to next section.
☐ Yes *If yes,* total number of sites_____ and complete appropriate section below.

Identify which of the following exception requirements applies to your laboratory operation.

Is this a non-profit or Federal, State or local government laboratory engaged in limited *(e.g., few types of tests)* public health testing and filing for a single certificate for multiple sites? ......☐ Yes   ☐ No *If yes,* list name, address and tests performed for each site below.

Is this a hospital with several laboratories at the same street address and under common direction that is filing for a single certificate for these locations? ....☐ Yes   ☐ No *If yes,* list name or department, location within hospital and specialty/subspecialty areas for each site below.

If additional space is needed, check here ____ and attach the additional information using the same format.

NAME AND ADDRESS / LOCATION	TESTS PERFORMED / SPECIALTY / SUBSPECIALTY
Name of laboratory or hospital department	
Address/location (number, street, location if applicable)	
City, State, ZIP — Telephone No. ( )	
Name of laboratory or hospital department	
Address/location (number, street, location if applicable)	
City, State, ZIP — Telephone No. ( )	
Name of laboratory or hospital department	
Address/location (number, street, location if applicable)	
City, State, ZIP — Telephone No. ( )	

FORM HCFA-116 (8-92)   Page 2 of 4

Health Care Financing Agency (HCFA) Form 116 (cont.)

VI. ACCREDITATION INFORMATION

Is your laboratory presently accredited by any private nonprofit organization ....☐ Yes   ☐ No

Accredited by: ☐ JCAHO   ☐ COLA   *If yes,* check all that apply:
☐ AOA   ☐ ASC
☐ AABB   ☐ ASHI
☐ CAP   ☐ Other *(specify)* _____

VII. WAIVED TESTING

Indicate total annual test volume for all waived tests performed. _____

VIII. NONWAIVED TESTING

If you perform testing other than or in addition to waived tests, complete the information below. If applying for one certificate for multiple sites, include information for all sites.

Place a check (√) in the box preceding each specialty/subspecialty in which the laboratory performs testing. Enter the test volume for the previous calendar year for each specialty. If you are a new laboratory or have added new specialties/subspecialties, for test volume, enter your estimated annual test volume. Do not include testing not subject to CLIA, waived tests, or tests run for quality control, quality assurance or proficiency testing when estimating total volume. Each profile, panel or group of tests usually performed simultaneously is counted as the total number of separate tests or procedures of which it is comprised. Calculations such as A/G ratio, MCH, MCHC and T_7 are an exception and should not be included in the total count. Examples: A chemistry profile consisting of 18 separate procedures is counted as 18 separate procedures. In the same manner, a CBC is counted as each individual measured (not calculated) analyte and as one test for the differential. For microbiology, susceptability testing is counted as one test per group of antiobiotics used to determine sensitivity for one organism.

If applying for certificate of accreditation, indicate name of current accrediting body beside applicable specialty/subspecialty.

SPECIALTY / SUBSPECIALTY	ACCREDITED PROGRAM	ANNUAL TEST VOLUME	SPECIALTY / SUBSPECIALTY	ACCREDITED PROGRAM	ANNUAL TEST VOLUME
☐ **Histocompatibility**			☐ **Hematology**		
☐ Transplant			☐ **Immunohematology**		
☐ Non-transplant			☐ ABO Group & Rh Group		
☐ **Microbiology**			☐ Antibody Detection (transfusion)		
☐ Bacteriology			☐ Antibody Detection (nontransfusion)		
☐ Mycobacteriology					
☐ Mycology			☐ Antibody Identification		
☐ Parasitology			☐ Compatibility Testing		
☐ Virology					
☐ Other			☐ Other		
☐ **Diagnostic Immunology**			☐ **Pathology**		
☐ Syphilis Serology			☐ Histopathology		
☐ General Immunology			☐ Oral Pathology		
☐ **Chemistry**			☐ Cytology		
☐ Routine					
☐ Urinalysis			☐ **Radiobioassay**		
☐ Endocrinology					
☐ Toxicology			☐ **Clinical Cytogenetics**		
☐ Other			**TOTAL ANNUAL TEST VOLUME**		

Health Care Financing Agency (HCFA) Form 116 (cont.)

IX. TYPE OF CONTROL	X. TYPE OF OWNERSHIP

Enter the appropriate two digit code from the list below _____ ____ *(enter only one code)*

Voluntary Nonprofit
01 Religious Affiliation
02 Private
03 Other

For Profit
04 Proprietary

Government
05 City
06 County
07 State
08 Federal
09 Other Government

Enter the appropriate two digit code from the list below _____ ____ *(enter only one code)*

01 Sole Proprietorship
02 Partnership
03 Corporation
04 Other *(specify)*

_____

XI. DIRECTOR AFFILIATION WITH OTHER LABORATORIES

If the primary director of this laboratory serves as primary director for laboratories that are separately certified, please complete the following:

NAME OF LABORATORY	ADDRESS	CLIA IDENTIFICATION NUMBER

XII. INDIVIDUALS INVOLVED IN LABORATORY TESTING

Indicate the total number of individuals involved in laboratory testing (directing, supervising, consulting or testing). Do not include individuals who only collect specimens or perform clerical duties. For nonwaived testing, only count an individual one time, at the highest laboratory position in which they function. (Example Pathologist serves as director, technical supervisor and general supervisor. This individual would only be counted once (under director)).

A. Waived TOTAL
  No. of Individuals _____

B. Nonwaived TOTAL No. of Individuals _____
            Director _____   Technical supervisor _____
   Clinical consultant _____   General supervisor _____
   Technical consultant _____   Testing personnel _____

ATTENTION: READ THE FOLLOWING CAREFULLY BEFORE SIGNING APPLICATION

ANY PERSON WHO INTENTIONALLY VIOLATES ANY REQUIREMENT OF SECTION 353 OF THE PUB-LIC HEALTH SERVICE ACT AS AMENDED OR ANY REGULATION PROMULGATED THEREUNDER SHALL BE IMPRISONED FOR NOT MORE THAN ONE YEAR OR FINED UNDER TITLE 18, UNITED STATES CODE OR BOTH, EXCEPT THAT IF THE CONVICTION IS FOR A SECOND OR SUBSEQUENT VIOLATION OF SUCH A REQUIREMENT SUCH PERSON SHALL BE IMPRISONED FOR NOT MORE THAN 3 YEARS OR FINED IN ACCORDANCE WITH TITLE 18, UNITED STATES CODE OR BOTH.

CONSENT: THE APPLICANT HEREBY AGREES THAT SUCH LABORATORY IDENTIFIED HEREIN WILL BE OPERATED IN ACCORDANCE WITH APPLICABLE STANDARDS FOUND NECESSARY BY THE SECRETARY OF HEALTH AND HUMAN SERVICES TO CARRY OUT THE PURPOSES OF SECTION 353 OF THE PUBLIC HEALTH SERVICE ACT AS AMENDED. THE APPLICANT FURTHER AGREES TO PERMIT THE SECRETARY, OR ANY FEDERAL OFFICER OR EMPLOYEE DULY DESIGNATED BY THE SECRETARY, TO INSPECT THE LABORATORY AND ITS OPERATIONS AND PERTINENT RECORDS AT ANY REASONABLE TIME.

SIGNATURE OF OWNER/AUTHORIZED REPRESENTATIVE OF LABORATORY *(sign in ink)*	DATE
last *first* *MI*	

FORM HCFA-116 (8-92)

Page 4 of 4

Health Care Financing Agency (HCFA) Form 116 (cont.)

PATIENT TEST REQUISITION AND REPORT

Patient Name:_____   ID # :_____

Address:_____   Telephone:_____

Date/Time Drawn:_____   Initials:_____

Date/Time Completed:_____   Initials:_____

Health Care Provider:_____   Address:_____

TEST	RESULT	NORMALS	COMMENT
glucose	_____	*76–115 mg/dL	_____
total cholesterol	_____	<200 mg/dL	_____
triglycerides	_____	<250 mg/dL	_____
HDL	_____	≥35 mg/dL	_____
calculated LDL	_____	<130 mg/dL	_____
glycosylated hemoglobin	_____	<7 mg%	_____

* Normal glucose for a fasting adult.

Enter "TNP" if the test was not performed.

Place in the patient's file.

Test Requisition and Report Form

CONTROL ___Low___   MEAN _____   MIN. _____   MAX. _____

Date	1	2	3	4	5	6	7	8	9	10	11	12	13	14	15	16	17	18	19	20	21	22	23	24	25	26	27	28	29	30	31
Tech																															
Value																															
Max																															
X																															
Min																															

CONTROL ___High___   MEAN _____   MIN. _____   MAX. _____

Date	1	2	3	4	5	6	7	8	9	10	11	12	13	14	15	16	17	18	19	20	21	22	23	24	25	26	27	28	29	30	31
Tech																															
Value																															
Max																															
X																															
Min																															

Self Chk

DATE   CORRECTIVE ACTION   TECH

_____

_____

REAGENT/NAME LOT # _____   EXP DATE _____

Instructions for Use:

1. Provide the acceptable control values as established by the manufacturer or in departmental policy. Transfer these values to the max/min grid and establish a scale for plotting data.
2. For each analysis performed, indicate the person performing the analysis and the value obtained in the initial and value rows, respectively.
3. Plot the value obtained in the grid using the scale established for the equipment or procedure being analyzed.
4. If the result was obtained from the equipment's self-checking feature, check the appropriate box.
5. Record the lot and expiration date of the reagent used, if any.
6. Explain any corrective action taken. Include date and initials.

Example Quality Control Chart

INSTRUMENT MAINTENANCE LOG

CHOLESTECH L-D-X®

SERIAL NUMBER _____

Date	Initials	Optics Check	Other (describe)

Example Instrument Maintenance Log

REFRIGERATOR TEMPERATURE LOG

REFRIGERATOR ID _____

ACCEPTABLE RANGE 2–8°C

Date	Initials	Temp.	Actions

Example Refrigerator Temperature Log

PERSONNEL TRAINING LOG

NAME_____

Date	Employee Signature	Trainer's Signature	Training Received (add as needed)
BLOODBORNE PATHOGEN EXPOSURE CONTROL PLAN			
			Bloodborne pathogens standards
			Universal precautions
			Protective equipment
			Accidental exposure procedures
LABORATORY OPERATIONS			
			Finger stick procedure
			Instrument operation & maintenance
			Quality control procedures
			Record-keeping procedures
			Proficiency testing (if applicable)
ANNUAL UPDATES			
			Bloodborne Pathogens Exposure Control Plan
			Laboratory Operations

Original: Facility Copy
Duplicate: Personnel File

Example Personnel Training Log

EXPOSURE REPORT

Postexposure Evaluation and Follow-up

Employee Name: _____

Social Security Number: _____

Date of Exposure: _____

Date Report Filled Out: _____

Describe the circumstances of the exposure:

What was the route of exposure?

List names of witnesses:

Describe HBV and HIV status of source patient, if known:

Describe any medical follow-up:

Copy to: Personnel File

Exposure Report

Patient Consent or Refusal for
HIV and HBV Infectivity Testing

Patient Name: _____

Date: _____

I understand that health care facilities are required by law to attempt to obtain consent for human immunodeficiency virus (HIV) and hepatitis B virus (HBV) infectivity testing each time a health care worker is exposed to the blood or bodily fluids OF ANY PATIENT. I understand that a health care worker has been accidentally exposed to my blood or bodily fluids and that testing for HIV and HBV infectivity is requested. I am not required to give my consent, but if I do, my blood will be tested for these viruses at no expense to me.

I have been informed that this test can produce a false positive result when an HIV antibody is not present and that follow-up tests may be required.

I understand that the results of these tests will be kept confidential and will only be released to medical personnel directly responsible for my care and treatment, to the exposed health care worker for his or her medical benefit only, and to others only as required by law.

I hereby consent to: I hereby refuse consent to:

❑ HIV testing   ❑ HIV testing

❑ HBV testing   ❑ HBV testing

Signature: _____

(If signed by someone other than patient, please explain relationship.)

HIV and HBV Testing Consent Form

PREGNANCY WAIVER FORM

NAME: _____

SOCIAL SECURITY NUMBER: _____

    I understand that due to my risk of occupational exposure to blood I may be placing my child at risk of acquiring hepatitis B virus (HBV) and human immunodeficiency virus (HIV) infections. I have been given the opportunity to stop working with blood. However, I have decided to continue working in situations that may result in exposure to blood. If in the future I reconsider my decision and I am still pregnant, I will be given the opportunity of not working in an area that requires exposure to blood.

_____   _____
Signature   Date

_____   _____
Witness' Signature   Date

_____
Witness' Name (Print)

Pregnancy Waiver Form

HEPATITIS B VACCINATION WAIVER FORM

NAME: _____

SOCIAL SECURITY NUMBER: _____

I understand that due to my risk of occupational exposure to blood I may be placing myself at risk of acquiring hepatitis B virus (HBV) infection. I have been given the opportunity by my employer, at no expense to myself, to receive the hepatitis B vaccination series. However, I have decided not to receive the hepatitis B vaccination series. If in the future, I reconsider my decision, I will be given the opportunity to receive the hepatitis B vaccination series at no cost to me.

_____
Signature   Date

_____
Witness' Signature   Date

_____
Witness' Name (Print)

Hepatitis B Vaccination Waiver Form

Content

- ❑ scientifically accurate
- ❑ unbiased in content and tone
- ❑ sufficiently specific and comprehensive
- ❑ presented in an understandable format that is readily comprehensible to consumers
- ❑ timely and up-to-date
- ❑ useful

Readability (Written Materials)

- ❑ sixth- through eighth-grade reading level (written materials)

Understandability

- ❑ appropriate use of medical terms
- ❑ avoidance of jargon

Appearance

Written Materials

- ❑ ≥10 point type (≥14 points for materials for elderly patients)
- ❑ avoids ornate typefaces or italics
- ❑ important information is in boldface type or in a box
- ❑ uppercase and lowercase lettering is used
- ❑ capitalization of entire words (MEDICA-TION) is avoided
- ❑ adequate space between letters, lines, and paragraphs
- ❑ line length approximately 40 letters long
- ❑ good contrast between ink and paper colors (black, dark blue, or brown ink on pale yellow or white paper is best)
- ❑ printed on uncoated paper
- ❑ short paragraphs and bullet points used

Audiovisual Materials

- ❑ appealing presentation
- ❑ avoidance of overdone graphics
- ❑ appropriate language level

Checklist for evaluating written, audio, and audiovisual patient education materials

Written Patient Education Materials Ordering/Tracking Form

Supplier	Material Title	Inventory Level	Quantity Ordered	Date Ordered	Quantity Received	Date Received	Cost

Educational Materials Ordering and Tracking Form

Pharmacist's Patient Database Form

Original Date:_____
Date updated:_____
Date updated:_____
Date updated:_____

Demographic and Administrative Information

Name:	Social Security #:
Address:	
Health Care Provider's Name	Health Care Provider's Phone
Work Phone: Home Phone:	Date of Birth:
Race:	Gender:
Religion:	Occupation:
Health Insurer:	Subscriber #:
Primary Card Holder:	Drug Benefit: ❑ yes ❑ no copay: $_____

Current Symptoms

Past Medical History	Acute and Current Medical Problems
	1.
	2.
	3.
	4.
	5.
	6.
	7.
	8.

Family/Social/Economic History	Personal Limitations
Cost of medications per month $_____	

Allergies/Intolerances		Social Drug Use
❑ No known drug allergies		Alcohol
Medication	Reaction	Caffeine
		Tobacco
		Pregnancy/Breastfeeding Status
		❑ Pregnant (due _____) ❑ Breastfeeding

Diet	Routine Exercise/Recreation	Daily Activities/Timing
❑ Low salt		
❑ Low fat		
❑ Diabetic		
Timing of meals:		

Pharmacist's Patient Database Form

Patient Name: _____

Current Prescription Medication Regimen

Name/Dose/Strength/Route	Schedule/ Frequency of Use	Indication	Start Date (and stop date if applicable)	Prescriber	Adherence Issues/Efficacy

Current Nonprescription Medication Regimen (OTC, herbal, homeopathic, nutritional, etc.)

Name/Dose/Strength/Route	Schedule/ Frequency of Use	Indication	Start Date (and stop date if applicable)	Prescriber	Adherence Issues/Efficacy

Pharmacist's Patient Database Form (cont.)

Patient Name: _____

Physical Assessment/Laboratory Data—Initial/Follow-up

Date					
Height					
Weight					
Temp					
BP					
Pulse					
Respirations					
Peak Flow					
FBG					
R. Glucose					
HgbA$_{1C}$					
T. Chol.					
LDL					
HDL					
TG					
INR					
BUN					
Cr					
ALT					
AST					
Alk Phos					

Drug Serum Concentrations

Date					

Notes:

Pharmacist's Patient Database Form (cont.)

Patient Name: _____

Risk Assessment/Preventive Measures/Quality of Life

Cardiovascular Risk Assessment		
male > 45 years old	1	
female > 55 years old or female < 55 with history of ovarectomy not taking estrogen replacement	1	
Definite MI or sudden death before age 55 year in father or male first-degree relative or before 65 year in mother or female first-degree relative	1	
current cigarette smoking	1	
hypertension	1	
diabetes mellitus	1	
HDL cholesterol < 35 mg/dl	1	
HDL cholesterol > 60 mg/dl	-1	
	Total:	

Is patient at risk for complications of current conditions? ❏ Yes   ❏ No
Specify:

Preventive Measures for Adults H = has been done R = patient refuses X = not applicable		Date				
Women						
Pap Smear/pelvic	Annually 19+					
Mammogram	Every 1-2Y 40-49; annually 50+					
Men						
Rectal/prostate	Annually 50+					
All Patients						
Total/HDL-C	Every 5Y 19+					
Home Fecal Occult Blood Test	Annually					
Immunizations						
Td	Every 10Y					
Influenza	Every fall*					
Pneumovax	Once*					

* if indicated

Quality of life issues

Pharmacist's Patient Database Form (cont.)

Ambulatory Therapy Assessment Worksheet (ATAW)

Patient
Pharmacist
Date

Correlation Between Drug Therapy and Medical Problems

ASSESSMENT	PRESENCE OF PROBLEM*	COMMENTS/NOTES
Any drugs without a medical indication? Any unidentified medications? Any untreated medical conditions? Do they require drug therapy?	1. A problem exists. 2. More information is needed for determination. 3. No problem exists or an intervention is not needed.	

Appropriate Therapy

ASSESSMENT	PRESENCE OF PROBLEM*	COMMENTS/NOTES
Comparative efficacy of chosen medication(s)? Relative safety of chosen medication(s)? Is medication on formulary? Is nondrug therapy appropriately used (e.g., diet and exercise)? Is therapy achieving desired goals or outcomes? Is therapy tailored to this patient (e.g., age, comorbid conditions, and living/working environment)?	1. A problem exists. 2. More information is needed for determination. 3. No problem exists or an intervention is not needed.	

Drug Regimen

ASSESSMENT	PRESENCE OF PROBLEM*	COMMENTS/NOTES
Are dose and dosing regimen appropriate and/or within usual therapeutic range and/or modified for patient factors? Appropriateness of PRN medications (prescribed or taken that way) Is route/dosage form/mode of administration appropriate, length or course of therapy considering efficacy, safety, convenience, patient limitations, length or course of therapy, and cost?	1. A problem exists. 2. More information is needed for determination. 3. No problem exists or an intervention is not needed.	

*Problem denotes any pharmacotherapeutic or related health care problem.

Ambulatory Therapy Assessment Worksheet (ATAW)

Therapeutic Duplication

ASSESSMENT	PRESENCE OF PROBLEM*	COMMENTS/NOTES
Any therapeutic duplications?	1. A problem exists. 2. More information is needed for determination. 3. No problem exists or an intervention is not needed.	

Drug Allergy or Intolerance

ASSESSMENT	PRESENCE OF PROBLEM*	COMMENTS/NOTES
Allergy or intolerance to any medications (or chemically related medications) currently being taken? Is patient using a method to alert health care providers of the allergy/intolerance or serious health problem?	1. A problem exists. 2. More information is needed for determination. 3. No problem exists or an intervention is not needed.	

Adverse Drug Events

ASSESSMENT	PRESENCE OF PROBLEM*	COMMENTS/NOTES
Are symptoms or medical problems drug induced? What is the likelihood the problem is drug related?	1. A problem exists. 2. More information is needed for determination. 3. No problem exists or an intervention is not needed.	

Interactions: Drug-Drug, Drug-Disease, Drug-Nutrient, Drug–Laboratory Test

ASSESSMENT	PRESENCE OF PROBLEM*	COMMENTS/NOTES
Any drug-drug interactions? Clinical significance? Any relative or absolute contraindications given patient characteristics and current/past disease states? Any drug-nutrient interactions? Clinical significance? Any drug-laboratory test interactions? Clinical significance?	1. A problem exists. 2. More information is needed for determination. 3. No problem exists or an intervention is not needed.	

*Problem denotes any pharmacotherapeutic or related health care problem.

Ambulatory Therapy Assessment Worksheet (ATAW) (cont.)

Social or Recreational Drug Use

ASSESSMENT	PRESENCE OF PROBLEM*	COMMENTS/NOTES
Is current use of social drugs problematic? Are symptoms related to sudden withdrawal or discontinuation of social drugs?	1. A problem exists. 2. More information is needed for determination. 3. No problem exists or an intervention is not needed.	

Financial Impact

ASSESSMENT	PRESENCE OF PROBLEM*	COMMENTS/NOTES
Is therapy cost-effective? Does cost of therapy represent a financial hardship for the patient?	1. A problem exists. 2. More information is needed for determination. 3. No problem exists or an intervention is not needed.	

Patient Knowledge of Therapy

ASSESSMENT	PRESENCE OF PROBLEM*	COMMENTS/NOTES
Does patient understand the role of his/her medication(s), how to take it, and potential side effects? Would patient benefit from education tools (e.g., written patient education sheets, wallet cards, or reminder package?) Does the patient understand the role of nondrug therapy?	1. A problem exists. 2. More information is needed for determination. 3. No problem exists or an intervention is not needed.	

Adherence

ASSESSMENT	PRESENCE OF PROBLEM*	COMMENTS/NOTES
Is there a problem with nonadherence to drug or nondrug therapy (e.g., diet and exercise)? Are there barriers to adherence or factors hindering the achievement of therapeutic efficacy?	1. A problem exists. 2. More information is needed for determination. 3. No problem exists or an intervention is not needed.	

*Problem denotes any pharmacotherapeutic or related health care problem.

Ambulatory Therapy Assessment Worksheet (ATAW) (cont.)

Self-Monitoring

ASSESSMENT	PRESENCE OF PROBLEM*	COMMENTS/NOTES
Does patient perform appropriate self-monitoring? (e.g., peak flow and blood glucose) Is correct technique employed? Is self-monitoring performed consistently, at appropriate times, and with appropriate frequency?	1. A problem exists. 2. More information is needed for determination. 3. No problem exists or an intervention is not needed.	

Risks and Quality of Life Impacts

ASSESSMENT	PRESENCE OF PROBLEM*	COMMENTS/NOTES
Is patient at risk for complications with an existing disease state (i.e., risk factor assessment)? Is patient on track for preventive measures (e.g., immunizations, mammograms, prostate exams, eye exams)? Is therapy adversely impacting patient's quality of life? How so?	1. A problem exists. 2. More information is needed for determination. 3. No problem exists or an intervention is not needed.	

*Problem denotes any pharmacotherapeutic or related health care problem.

Ambulatory Therapy Assessment Worksheet (ATAW) (cont.)

Ambulatory Pharmacist's Care Plan

Patient _____

Pharmacist _____

Date _____

DATE IDENTIFIED	PROBLEM (TPL)	PHARMACOTHERAPEUTIC AND RELATED HEALTH CARE GOAL	RECOMMENDATIONS FOR THERAPY	MONITORING PARAMETER(S)	DESIRED ENDPOINT(S)	MONITORING FREQUENCY

Ambulatory Pharmacist's Care Plan Form

PHARMACIST'S CARE PLAN AMBULATORY MONITORING WORKSHEET (AMW)

Patient _____

Pharmacist _____
Date _____

Pharmaco-theropeutic Goal	Monitoring Parameter	Desired Endpoint	Monitoring Frequency	Date								

Pharmacist's Care Plan Ambulatory Monitoring Worksheet (AMW)

LIABILITY WAIVER FORM

I hereby consent to have blood samples drawn for the purpose of screening. I understand that there may be some discomfort, bruising, bleeding, or swelling at the puncture site and surrounding tissue, and that it may become infected. If signs of infection are seen (redness, swelling, warmth, pain, or pus), I will seek medical care.

I hereby release _____, their affiliates, directors, officers, employees, successors, and assigns from any and all liability arising from or in any way connected with this blood drawing for my measurements or from the data derived therefrom. I understand that:

I should not participate in this test if I suffer from any bleeding disorder or similar condition.

The data derived from this test are to be considered preliminary only and must be confirmed with additional tests. We advise that you review the results of this test with your physician.

Date:_____

Name:_____

Signature:_____

Example Liability Waiver Form

Patient Screening Questionnaire

I. Type of Screening

Please put a check (√) next to the screening tests listed below that you wish to have performed:

_____ blood glucose
_____ total cholesterol
_____ HDL cholesterol
_____ total cholesterol/HDL cholesterol ratio
_____ lipid profile
_____ blood pressure

II. Patient Information

Date: _____
Name: _____
Address:_____
_____
Home Phone:_____
Office Phone:_____
Date of Birth:_____ Age:_____
Name of Health Insurer:_____
Health Ins. Card #_____
Social Security #: _____
Primary Care Physician's Name: _____
Phone:_____
Specialist Physician's Name:_____
Phone:_____
Date and time of last food or beverage_____

III. Medical History

Please put a check (√) next to the statements that are true:

_____I have high blood pressure.
_____I take medication for high blood pressure.
_____I have diabetes.
_____I take medication for diabetes.
_____I have high cholesterol.
_____I take medication for high cholesterol.
_____I have had a stroke.
_____I have had heart bypass surgery
_____I have had a heart attack.

IV. Heart Disease Risk Factors

Please put a check (√) next to the statements which are true:

_____I have high blood pressure.
_____I have diabetes.
_____I smoke cigarettes.
_____I am a male over the age of 45.
_____I am a female over the age of 55.
_____I am a female less than 55 years old, I have had my ovaries removed, and I am not taking estrogen therapy.
_____My father or brother died of a heart attack before age 55.
_____My mother or sister died of a heart attack before age 65.
_____I have had chest pain (angina).
_____I have had heart bypass surgery.

I certify to the best of my knowledge the above information is true.

_____
(signature)

Patient Screening Questionnaire

DIABETES SCREENING RESULTS

Diabetes is a condition in which the body cannot use sugar (also referred to as glucose) properly. There are about 14 million people with diabetes in the United States. Half of them have not yet been diagnosed. It is important to diagnose diabetes early. Early detection and treatment may limit some of the long-term complications of diabetes. These include vision loss, kidney disease, heart disease, nerve damage, and damage to the blood vessels in the legs, feet, and hands.

Your chance of developing diabetes is greater if you:
- are overweight
- have a family history of diabetes
- are a woman who delivered babies weighing over 9 pounds or had diabetes during pregnancy
- are African American
- are Hispanic
- are a Native American

Many symptoms can occur if a patient has diabetes. Each patient will have different symptoms. Some patients have severe symptoms while others have no symptoms at all. Some symptoms of diabetes include:
- more frequent urination
- increased thirst
- tiredness
- weakness
- dizziness
- increased hunger
- slow wound healing
- more frequent infections

In a person without diabetes the blood glucose level is normally 60–126 mg/dl (milligrams of glucose in each deciliter of blood). Results above 126 mg/dl are considered high and measurements below 60 mg/dl are considered low. A single high reading does not mean you have diabetes, but you should see your doctor for further evaluation.

Your blood glucose is: _____

Date: _____

Time: _____

Date last food or beverage was consumed: _____

Time last food or beverage was consumed: _____

Diabetes Screening Results Form

BLOOD PRESSURE SCREENING RESULTS

The heart is a muscle that pumps blood through the blood vessels in the body. When the heart beats, it squeezes blood into the blood vessels and creates pressure in them. This pressure is needed to circulate blood through the entire body. The heart beats 60–100 times each minute and rests between each beat.

Blood pressure is highest when the heart beats and lowest when the heart rests. Therefore, a patient really has two levels of blood pressure: an upper one when the heart is beating and a lower one when the heart is resting. The higher pressure is called the systolic pressure. The lower pressure is referred to as the diastolic pressure. The systolic blood pressure is important because it tells the maximum amount of pressure placed on the blood vessels. The diastolic pressure tells the minimum amount of pressure placed on the blood vessels.

Both the diastolic and systolic levels are recorded when your blood pressure is measured. For example, if your blood pressure reading is recorded as 110/85 (110 over 85), the top number (110) is the systolic pressure and the bottom number (85) is the diastolic pressure. Blood pressure is measured in the units "mmHg" (millimeters of mercury).

When someone's blood pressure is higher than the desirable range, they have hypertension. *Hyper* means high and *tension* refers to pressure. For most adults a blood pressure reading above 140/90 mmHg is considered higher than the desirable range. Adults who have diabetes or kidney damage have a lower desirable range.

In about 90% of people with hypertension, the cause is unknown. Several factors seem to increase the risk for developing hypertension. These include heredity; male gender; older age; black race; obesity; sensitivity to sodium; heavy alcohol consumption; the use of certain medications such as decongestants, nonsteroidal anti-inflammatory agents, and products containing sodium; smoking; and an inactive lifestyle.

Over 60 million Americans have hypertension. In general, hypertension has no symptoms, but if untreated it can lead to serious complications, such as stroke, heart attacks, and heart failure. Some patients may complain of headache or changes in vision such as blurred vision, but most people are not aware they have hypertension until they have their blood pressure measured.

A single high reading does not mean you have hypertension, but you should see your doctor for further evaluation.

Your blood pressure today is:_____

Date: _____

Time: _____

Blood Pressure Screening Results Form

CHOLESTEROL SCREENING RESULTS

Cholesterol is a fat-like substance found in all your body's cells. Cholesterol is used to make cell membranes and certain hormones in your body. Problems may occur when you have too much cholesterol.

Cholesterol comes from two sources. It is produced normally in your body and also comes from certain foods in your diet. Cholesterol travels throughout the body to where it is needed. Because cholesterol is made up of fat, it cannot travel through the blood by itself (fat cannot mix with water). Instead it must be transported to and from cells by special carriers called lipoproteins. There are several types of lipoproteins, but the ones we are most concerned about are low-density lipoprotein (LDL) and high-density lipoprotein (HDL).

LDL is called "bad" cholesterol because it sticks to the inside wall of blood vessels, increasing the chance of developing coronary heart disease. HDL cholesterol, or "good" cholesterol, rescues LDL that is stuck on the blood vessel wall and returns it to the liver.

Triglycerides are a type of fat found in lipoproteins. Various lipoproteins contain different amounts of triglycerides. The triglyceride level in the blood is highest right after eating a meal containing fat.

If your cholesterol level is too high, LDL cholesterol will deposit in the blood vessels that supply the heart muscle with blood and oxygen and narrow the blood vessels. This is referred to as coronary artery disease. Eventually the blood vessels narrow so much that the blood supply is decreased. When the blood supply decreases, the heart muscle does not receive enough oxygen and is damaged. A heart attack occurs when there is damage to the heart muscle.

In general, total blood cholesterol should be less than 200 mg/dl (milligrams of cholesterol per deciliter of blood). If the total cholesterol is above 200 mg/dl, it is considered too high.

A single high reading does not mean you have high cholesterol, but you should see your doctor for further evaluation. You may need to have another test of your cholesterol which tells you how much "good" and "bad" cholesterol you have in your blood. This test is called a lipid profile.

Your total cholesterol is: _____

Date: _____

Time: _____

Date last food or beverage was consumed: _____

Time last food or beverage was consumed: _____

Cholesterol Screening Results Form

CHOLESTEROL SCREENING RESULTS (FOR FULL LIPID PROFILE)

Cholesterol is a fat-like substance found in all your body's cells. Cholesterol is used to make cell membranes and certain hormones in your body. Problems may occur when you have too much cholesterol.

Cholesterol comes from two sources. It is produced normally in your body and also comes from certain foods in your diet. Cholesterol travels throughout the body to where it is needed. Because cholesterol is made up of fat, it cannot travel through the blood by itself (fat cannot mix with water). Instead it must be transported to and from cells by special carriers called lipoproteins. There are several types of lipoproteins, but the ones we are most concerned about are low-density lipoprotein (LDL) and high-density lipoprotein (HDL).

LDL is called "bad" cholesterol because it sticks to the inside wall of blood vessels, increasing the chance of developing coronary heart disease. HDL cholesterol, or "good" cholesterol, rescues LDL that is stuck on the blood vessel wall and returns it to the liver.

Triglycerides are a type of fat found in lipoproteins. Various lipoproteins contain different amounts of triglycerides. The triglyceride level in the blood is highest right after eating a meal containing fat.

If your cholesterol level is too high, LDL cholesterol will deposit in the blood vessels that supply the heart muscle with blood and oxygen and narrow the blood vessels. This is referred to as coronary artery disease. Eventually the blood vessels narrow so much that the blood supply is decreased. When the blood supply decreases, the heart muscle does not receive enough oxygen and is damaged. A heart attack occurs when there is damage to the heart muscle.

In general, total blood cholesterol should be less than 200 mg/dl (milligrams of cholesterol per deciliter of blood). If the total cholesterol is above 200 mg/dl, it is considered too high.

The triglyceride level in the blood should be less than 250 mg/dl.

The HDL cholesterol level should be more than 35 mg/dl.

The recommended goal for LDL cholesterol depends on two criteria. The first is the presence of coronary artery disease and the second is the number of coronary heart disease risk factors.

Risk factors for coronary heart disease are conditions that increase a person's chance of developing coronary heart disease. These risk factors include:

- being a male over the age of 45
- being a female over the age of 55 OR being a female under the age of 55 who is not taking hormone replacement therapy after having both ovaries removed.
- having a male sibling or parent who died of a heart attack or had a heart attack before age 55
- having a female parent or sibling who died of a heart attack or had a heart attack before age 65
- smoking cigarettes
- having high blood pressure
- having diabetes
- having a low HDL cholesterol (less than 35 mg/dl [milligrams of HDL cholesterol in each deciliter of blood])

Cholesterol Screening Results (for Full Lipid Profile) Form

If you have coronary heart disease, your LDL cholesterol should be less than 100 mg/dl.

If you do not have coronary artery disease but have two or more risk factors for coronary heart disease, your LDL cholesterol should be less than 130 mg/dl.

If you do not have coronary heart disease and have less than two risk factors for coronary heart disease, your LDL cholesterol should be less than 160 mg/dl.

A single high reading does not mean you have high cholesterol, but you should see your doctor for further evaluation.

Your total cholesterol is: _____

Your HDL cholesterol is:_____

Your LDL cholesterol is:_____

Your triglycerides are:_____

Date: _____

Time: _____

Date last food or beverage was consumed: _____

Time last food or beverage was consumed: _____

Cholesterol Screening Results (for Full Lipid Profile) Form (continued)

At your appointment on _____,
we will measure your fasting blood glucose
level. A fasting measurement is the most
consistent blood glucose level. If you are
taking medicine for diabetes, a fasting level
helps us evaluate how well your medicine
works overnight. Please observe the following
directions to ensure the results are accurate:

THE DAY BEFORE THE TEST

After _____, (time) do not
eat or drink anything except water.

THE DAY OF THE TEST

Do not eat or drink anything except
water until after the test is performed.

DO NOT take your diabetes medication
(oral agent and/or insulin) until after the test
is performed.

Take all other medications as directed.

If you have any questions, please contact
your pharmacist at _____.

**Fasting Blood Glucose Screening Instruction
Form**

At your appointment on _____,
we will measure your fasting lipid profile. This
test will allow us to measure your LDL
cholesterol, HDL cholesterol, triglycerides,
and total cholesterol level. Because some of
these values are affected by food, it is important that you observe the following directions
to be sure the results are accurate:

THE DAY BEFORE THE TEST

After _____, (time) do not
eat or drink anything except water.

THE DAY OF THE TEST

Do not eat or drink anything except
water until after the test is performed.

Take all of your medications as usual.

If you have any questions, please contact
your pharmacist at _____.

Fasting Lipid Profile Instruction Form

At your appointment on _____, we will measure your blood pressure. Please observe the following directions to be sure the results are accurate:

THE DAY OF THE TEST

Take all of your medications as directed, including your blood pressure medication.

Wear clothing that does not limit the blood flow in the arms when the blood pressure measurement is performed. (Restrictive clothing can falsely elevate the blood pressure).

Arrive at least 10 minutes early so that you can be seated comfortably and rest before the measurement. (Physical activity and stress can falsely elevate the blood pressure).

30 MINUTES BEFORE THE APPOINTMENT

1. Do not drink beverages that contain caffeine (such as coffee, tea, or soft drinks) 30 minutes before the appointment. (Caffeine can falsely elevate blood pressure.)

2. Do not use tobacco products 30 minutes before the appointment. This includes cigarettes, cigars, and chewing tobacco. (Nicotine can falsely elevate blood pressure.)

If you have any questions, please contact your pharmacist at _____.

Blood Pressure Screening Instruction Form

PATIENT RELEASE STATEMENT

I understand that my Good Health Pharmacy pharmacist will be working to help me improve and maintain my health through a better understanding of my health problems and helping me make the most effective use of my medications. As part of this process, Good Health Pharmacy will provide health-related information about me and the services I have received to my physicians to keep them informed of my progress and will provide information necessary for billing to my insurance company.

I hereby authorize Good Health Pharmacy to release to my physician and insurance company, _____, all information and records related to the care I receive.

I understand that a portion of Good Health Pharmacy's service includes my giving a series of blood samples for the purpose of monitoring. There may be some discomfort, bruising, bleeding, or swelling at the puncture site and surrounding tissue, and it may become infected. If I see signs of infection (redness, swelling, warmth, pain, or pus), I will seek medical care from my physician.

I hereby release Good Health Pharmacy, their affiliates, directors, officers, employees, successors, and assigns from any and all liability arising from or in any way connected with this release of such information and with this blood drawing. I understand that I should not participate in these tests if I suffer from any bleeding disorder or similar condition.

Date:_____

Printed name: _____

Signature:_____

Patient Release Form

STATEMENT OF MEDICAL NECESSITY

Patient Name: _____ Date:_____

Address: _____

City: _____ State:_____ Zip: _____

Home Telephone:_____ Date of Birth: _____

Diagnosis (ICD-9) _____

Patient Problem(s): _____

_____

Requested Services   **(✓)**

• Comprehensive _____ self-management instruction   _____

• Self-management assessment   _____

• Home monitoring instruction

        • _____   _____

        • _____   _____

• Medication administration instruction (_____)   _____

• Medication regimen adherence   _____

Goals of service requested: _____

_____

Anticipated duration:_____

I consider these requested services to be a necessary part of the patient's care.

_____   _____

Physician's Signature   *Date*

Physician Name (print): _____

Practice Address: _____

Telephone: _____ UPIN/NPI: _____

Statement of Medical Necessity

PLEASE
DO NOT
STAPLE
IN THIS
AREA

HEALTH INSURANCE CLAIM FORM

PICA		PICA

1. MEDICARE MEDICAID CHAMPUS CHAMPVA GROUP FECA OTHER	1a. INSURED'S I.D. NUMBER (FOR PROGRAM IN ITEM 1)

1. MEDICARE (Medicare #) MEDICAID (Medicaid #) CHAMPUS (Sponsor's SSN) CHAMPVA (VA File #) GROUP HEALTH PLAN (SSN or ID) FECA BLK LUNG (SSN) OTHER (ID)   1a. INSURED'S I.D. NUMBER   (FOR PROGRAM IN ITEM 1)

2. PATIENT'S NAME (Last Name, First Name, Middle Initial)   3. PATIENT'S BIRTH DATE MM | DD | YY   SEX M   F   4. INSURED'S NAME (Last Name, First Name, Middle Initial)

5. PATIENT'S ADDRESS (No., Street)   6. PATIENT RELATIONSHIP TO INSURED   Self   Spouse   Child   Other   7. INSURED'S ADDRESS (No., Street)

CITY   STATE   8. PATIENT STATUS   Single   Married   Other   CITY   STATE

ZIP CODE   TELEPHONE (Include Area Code) (   )   Employed   Full-Time Student   Part-Time Student   ZIP CODE   TELEPHONE (INCLUDE AREA CODE) (   )

9. OTHER INSURED'S NAME (Last Name, First Name, Middle Initial)   10. IS PATIENT'S CONDITION RELATED TO: 11. INSURED'S POLICY GROUP OR FECA NUMBER

a. OTHER INSURED'S POLICY OR GROUP NUMBER   a. EMPLOYMENT? (CURRENT OR PREVIOUS)   YES   NO   a. INSURED'S DATE OF BIRTH MM | DD | YY   SEX M   F

b. OTHER INSURED'S DATE OF BIRTH MM | DD | YY   SEX M   F   b. AUTO ACCIDENT?   PLACE (State)   YES   NO   b. EMPLOYER'S NAME OR SCHOOL NAME

c. EMPLOYER'S NAME OR SCHOOL NAME   c. OTHER ACCIDENT?   YES   NO   c. INSURANCE PLAN NAME OR PROGRAM NAME

d. INSURANCE PLAN NAME OR PROGRAM NAME   10d. RESERVED FOR LOCAL USE   d. IS THERE ANOTHER HEALTH BENEFIT PLAN?   YES   NO   If yes, return to and complete item 9 a-d.

READ BACK OF FORM BEFORE COMPLETING & SIGNING THIS FORM.
12. PATIENT'S OR AUTHORIZED PERSON'S SIGNATURE I authorize the release of any medical or other information necessary to process this claim. I also request payment of government benefits either to myself or to the party who accepts assignment below.

SIGNED _____   DATE _____

13. INSURED'S OR AUTHORIZED PERSON'S SIGNATURE I authorize payment of medical benefits to the undersigned physician or supplier for services described below.

SIGNED _____

14. DATE OF CURRENT: MM | DD | YY   ILLNESS (First symptom) OR INJURY (Accident) OR PREGNANCY(LMP)   15. IF PATIENT HAS HAD SAME OR SIMILAR ILLNESS. GIVE FIRST DATE MM | DD | YY   16. DATES PATIENT UNABLE TO WORK IN CURRENT OCCUPATION FROM MM | DD | YY   TO MM | DD | YY

17. NAME OF REFERRING PHYSICIAN OR OTHER SOURCE   17a. I.D. NUMBER OF REFERRING PHYSICIAN   18. HOSPITALIZATION DATES RELATED TO CURRENT SERVICES FROM MM | DD | YY   TO MM | DD | YY

19. RESERVED FOR LOCAL USE   20. OUTSIDE LAB?   YES   NO $ CHARGES

21. DIAGNOSIS OR NATURE OF ILLNESS OR INJURY. (RELATE ITEMS 1,2,3 OR 4 TO ITEM 24E BY LINE)
1. ____ . ____   3. ____ . ____
2. ____ . ____   4. ____ . ____

22. MEDICAID RESUBMISSION CODE   ORIGINAL REF. NO.
23. PRIOR AUTHORIZATION NUMBER

24.	A DATE(S) OF SERVICE From To MM DD YY MM DD YY	B Place of Service	C Type of Service	D PROCEDURES, SERVICES, OR SUPPLIES (Explain Unusual Circumstances) CPT/HCPCS	MODIFIER	E DIAGNOSIS CODE	F $ CHARGES	G DAYS OR UNITS	H EPSDT Family Plan	I EMG	J COB	K RESERVED FOR LOCAL USE
1										
2										
3										
4										
5										
6										

25. FEDERAL TAX I.D. NUMBER   SSN EIN   26. PATIENT'S ACCOUNT NO.   27. ACCEPT ASSIGNMENT? (For govt. claims, see back)   YES   NO   28. TOTAL CHARGE $ 29. AMOUNT PAID $ 30. BALANCE DUE $

31. SIGNATURE OF PHYSICIAN OR SUPPLIER INCLUDING DEGREES OR CREDENTIALS (I certify that the statements on the reverse apply to this bill and are made a part thereof.)

SIGNED _____   DATE _____

32. NAME AND ADDRESS OF FACILITY WHERE SERVICES WERE RENDERED (If other than home or office)

33. PHYSICIAN'S, SUPPLIER'S BILLING NAME, ADDRESS, ZIP CODE & PHONE #

PIN#   GRP#

(APPROVED BY AMA COUNCIL ON MEDICAL SERVICE 8/88)   **PLEASE PRINT OR TYPE**   FORM HCFA-1500 (12-90) FORM OWCP-1500   FORM RRB-1500

Health Care Financing Agency (HCFA) Claim Form 1500

Case Study

APPENDIX

2

Case Study

Seven years ago, a large-staff model HMO (in excess of 300,000 lives), located in the Midwest of the United States, hired an innovative pharmacist to head its pharmacy department. With an existing staff of four clinical pharmacists, the recently hired head of pharmacy knew creating a successful place for the pharmacy department within the organization would require focus and dedication of the department and staff to meet any and all goals established as the outcomes criteria for a successful program. During the negotiations for the position, the new head of pharmacy sought an organizational structure that would allow access to the decision-makers in the health plan and would report directly to the chief operating officer of the HMO rather than through the medical officer. To compensate for the medical supervision necessary, he requested a one-half full-time employee (FTE) physician to work with the pharmacy department.

The following guiding principles, developed at the inception of the program, have focused the department on the areas of service that would prove beneficial to the organization and aid in the growth and success of the department:

- All services must have measurable financial outcomes.
- Any service provided must not compete with other providers within the organization.
- Any service must receive the support of the physician liaison and chief medical officer, to be initiated.
- Results would be analyzed and communicated to all interested parties, specifically senior management.

With these guiding principles, the initial program was designed to impact drug cost. Pharmacists were placed in the clinic with physicians and made available to help with initial prescribing, with the goal of making prescribing habits more clinical and cost-effective. The pharmacists were available for any consultation and earned the trust of the physicians one patient at a time. The goal was a realistic slowing of the growth of prescription costs, and it was quickly achieved.

From this program grew the establishment of pharmacist-run programs in anticoagulation therapy, cardiac therapy, and home care, with 17 clinical pharmacists staffing the initial program of consulting with physicians on patient drug use. There are currently 60 clinical pharmacists assisting other providers in the delivery of care to patients.

The programs were designed to improve care and be cost-effective. When the anticoagulation therapy program was established, the goal was to reduce hospitalizations by better control of therapy. The program was designed to make it easy for the patient and maximize the pharmacist's productivity. The patient could use any of 17 drawing stations, and the results were faxed to the pharmacist at a central location. The patient was then contacted by telephone and his or her therapy was adjusted accordingly. Ninety-five percent of the interventions were handled by telephone, creating a cost-effective program. There were other beneficial aspects of having such a program, which allowed for further growth. The program increased physician comfort with anticoagulation, improving the percentage of appropriate prescribing. The program then moved into protocols for use of low-molecular-weight heparin and has reduced hospitalizations further. The program now has 11 FTE clinical pharmacists providing service.

Continually marketing the success of the program to senior management and medical management, with the support of the physician staff, has been crucial in maintaining and growing programs. This has been accomplished with serious data collection and analysis. Continuous quality improvement has kept the department's focus on the guiding principles and, therefore, increased the role for pharmacists in the organization.